CRITICAL EPIDEMIOLOGY AND
THE PEOPLE'S HEALTH

Small Books, Big Ideas in Population Health
Nancy Krieger, Series Editor

CRITICAL EPIDEMIOLOGY AND THE PEOPLE'S HEALTH

Jaime Breilh

PROFESSOR AND EX-RECTOR
UNIVERSIDAD ANDINA SIMÓN
BOLÍVAR (UASB-E)
DIRECTOR OF THE CENTER FOR
RESEARCH AND EVALUATION OF
COLLECTIVE HEALTH
(CILABSALUD)

OXFORD
UNIVERSITY PRESS

Oxford University Press is a department of the University of Oxford. It furthers the University's objective of excellence in research, scholarship, and education by publishing worldwide. Oxford is a registered trade mark of Oxford University Press in the UK and certain other countries.

Published in the United States of America by Oxford University Press
198 Madison Avenue, New York, NY 10016, United States of America.

Library of Congress Cataloging-in-Publication Data
Names: Breilh, Jaime, author.
Title: Critical epidemiology and the people's health / Jaime Breilh.
Other titles: Small books with big ideas.
Description: New York, NY : Oxford University Press, 2021. |
Series: Small books, big ideas in population health |
Includes bibliographical references and index.
Identifiers: LCCN 2020017239 | ISBN 9780190492786 (hardback)
Subjects: MESH: Epidemiologic Methods | Social Medicine | Social
Determinants of Health | Health Equity
Classification: LCC RA651 | NLM WA 950 | DDC 614.4—dc23
LC record available at https://lccn.loc.gov/2020017239

DOI: 10.1093/med/9780190492786.001.0001

9 8 7 6 5 4 3 2 1

Printed by Integrated Books International, United States of America

And then, above all, there is the new arrival—the thinking that does not shy away from the horror of the world, the darkness, but looks it straight in the face, and thus passes over into a different kingdom, which is not the kingdom of darkness. This thinking asserts itself while wandering among illusions and lies, beyond truth as well as error. If a consciousness of ineluctability wins out, then we have nihilism and the confirmation of decline.

—LEFEBVRE (2014)

CONTENTS

CONTENTS

FOREWORD

Critical ideas for tumultuous times. As political, economic and social polarization and inequities within and between countries escalates, and the fast-growing climate crisis and environmental degradation accelerate (People's Health Movement 2017; Beckfield 2018; Friel 2019; Latour 2018; Krieger 2020), urgent need exists for clarity about causes of—and paths towards rectifying—rampant health injustices.

In epidemiology, as in all sciences, the ideas and questions animating the field necessarily engage with the very world that scientists inhabit and seek to understand—and their place within this world (Krieger 2011a; Felt et al 2017; Oreskes 2019). For epidemiologists and others concerned about the people's health and planetary health, analyzing who and what shapes population distributions of health is necessarily informed by diverse and contending philosophical and political worldviews, grounded in the intimately and inseparably political, social, biological, ecosystemic, and historically dynamic realities of life on our planet (Krieger 2011a, 2020; Felt et al 2017; Latour 2018).

Embracing, rather than obscuring, these debates has been a cardinal feature of Latin American critical epidemiology since its emergence in the 1970s (Breilh 1979, 2003, 2008, 2019; Laurell 1989, 203, 2018; Franco et al. 1991; Iriat et al. 2002; Tajer 2003).

Born in a context of opposition to authoritarian rule and military dictatorships, in countries with complex histories and struggles involving settler colonialism, imperialism, enslavement, and Indigenous populations, Latin American critical epidemiology, as part of the Latin American Social Medicine/Collective Health movement, has critically guided research and action regarding the societal determination of health (Breilh 1979, 2003, 2008, 2019; Laurell 1989, 2003, 2018; Franco et al. 1991; Iriat et al. 2002; Tajer 2003). For too long, however, the rich discussions of Latin American critical epidemiology have appeared in primarily in publications written in Spanish or Portuguese. They have not, with some notable exceptions (Barreto et al. 2001; Iriat et al. 2002; Krieger 2003, 2011a; Tajer 2003; Laurell 1989, 2003, 2018; Franco 2003; Yamada 2003; Waitzkin 2001, 2008, 2011; Breilh 2008, 2019; Cueto 2015; Birn et al. 2017; Birn and Muntaner 2019; Vasquez et al. 2019), been readily accessible to readers for whom English is their primary scientific language.

This new volume of the Oxford series *"Small Book, Big Ideas in Population Health"* (OUP 2020) accordingly deliberately features, in English, the work of Jaime Breilh, a longstanding incisive and influential proponent and practitioner of Latin American critical epidemiology (Breilh 1979, 2003, 2008, 2019; Franco et al 1991), whom I first met in the late 1980s. Publishing this volume is part of a lifelong commitment I made, early on in my work in public health, to connect progressive thinking about social justice and public health across the Americas (Krieger 1988, 2002, 2003, 2011b, 2015; Krieger et al. 2010). It is also part of my commitment, embodied in the ecosocial theory of disease distribution I first proposed in 1994 and have elaborated since, to weave together critical political, historical, biological, and ecological thinking into the ideas and practices of epidemiology and other population health sciences (Krieger 1994, 2001, 2011a, 2014, 2020).

I keenly recall one moment when I was a graduate student getting my master degree in epidemiology in the US in the early 1980s and I was in the library—and unexpectedly came across an article titled: "Mercury poisoning in Nicaragua: A case study of the export of environmental and occupational hazards by a multi-national corporation" (Hassan et al. 1981). Published in 1981, two years after the then progressive overthrow of the Somoza military dictatorship, the article appeared in the *International Journal of Health Services*, then a decade old. Its editor, Dr. Vicente Navarro, had left Spain in the 1960s in a context of opposition to the Franco dictatorship, and had many ties to progressive Latin American colleagues, as reflected in the journal's editorial board (Navarro 2020). The article vividly documented how the Somoza regime had suppressed knowledge about how an industrial plant had been poisoning its workers and other people and wildlife adjacent to and depending on the water of Lake Managua—and how this knowledge only became public, and thus actionable, following the regime's overthrow (Hassan et al. 1981). It offered an eye-opening glimpse of what critical Latin American insights could offer North Americans in our own work for health equity.

Breilh's analysis complements the foci of the series' first two books: *Political Sociology and The People's Health* (Beckfield 2018) and *Climate Change and The People's Health* (Friel 2019). Drawing on Latin American critical thinking and movements, his text seeks to illuminate, challenge, and transform the under-lying conceptual and ideological assumptions—and sociopolitical contexts—that inform contemporary epidemiological theories, knowledge, and practice.

Hence: in Chapter 1, Breilh introduces the historical trajectory and panorama of critical thought in Latin American Social Medicine/Collective Health and the intertwined sociopolitical and ecological contexts and crises giving rise to this work and rendering it more relevant than ever. In Chapter 2, he delineates the theoretical underpinnings of Latin American critical epidemiology and provides concrete empirical examples of its utility to guide critical research. In Chapter 3, he urges epidemiology specifically, and public health more generally, to incorporate transformative, transdisciplinary, and intercultural ideas and practices to improve collective health, building on the strengths of both critical scientific and Indigenous knowledge.

At a time when the North American and European English-language epidemiological literature is embroiled in seemingly narrow debates—albeit with far-reaching consequences—about conceptual and methodological approaches to causal inference (VanderWeele 2015; Krieger and Davey Smith 2016; Vandenbroucke et al. 2016; Schwartz et al. 2016; Galea and Hernán 2019; Robinson and Bailey 2019), Breilh's arguments may seem as if they come from another planet. But they are very much grounded in the terrestrial realities of life on Earth. For all peoples to thrive and planetary health to flourish, we would do well to learn from the critical insights of the Latin American critical epidemiology, as aptly synthesized by Jaime Breilh.

—Nancy Krieger (February 13, 2020)

ACKNOWLEDGMENTS

I am especially grateful to my dear colleague Nancy Krieger for her invitation to contribute to the *Small Books, Big Ideas in Population Health* series. Her kind appreciation of my work has given me the opportunity to present to the English-speaking audience a complete synthesis of cardinal pioneering elements of Latin American critical epidemiology. In addition to the honor of joining a distinguished group of authors, this has been an unparalleled opportunity to participate in the international debate on the new pathways for the epidemiological science. An important motivation for my enthusiasm was also the fact that the series is being produced in partnership with Oxford University Press (OUP), a prominent, well-renowned scientific publisher. I am especially grateful to Chad Zimmerman, former Clinical Medicine Editor at OUP, for endorsing my participation and suggesting that I provide a consistent panorama of my own ideas and Latin American contributions. More recently, Sarah Humphreville joined the OUP editorial staff; I thank her for her lucid and kind support. I express my gratitude to all three of them for their patience. The production of my book was involuntarily delayed because I had to assume my position as democratically elected rector of my university just when I started working on the book a couple years ago. This unexpected privilege and opportunity to serve my academic community and my country was an ethical imperative in crucial moments of the defense of superior education autonomy and the protection of the right to critical academic freedom.

In a lifetime dedicated to critical research and epistemological debate, I have met so many good, inspiring, and supportive people who supportedmy work, taught me so much, and gave me a hand at critical moments that it is not possible to list them all here. But I recognize and am especially thankful to all those who in recent years not only allowed me the time to prepare the materials of the book and the initial English texts but also persistently facilitated with their reflections and advice the difficult work of preparing in the English language an abridged version of complex epistemological, methodological, and practical elements of the contemporary debate on epidemiology and the nature of science.

I thank my intimate familiar circle: three generous, talented, conscious and strong women—Cristina, María Cristina, and María José, my beloved wife and two daughters—who have valued my work, helped polish it, and offered me their support in times of doubt. I also thank my dear grandchild and son-in-law, who kept close and supportive, even in the difficult days of my struggle as rector.

I am thankful to my university and my colleagues in the Health Science Area for their participation in the rounds of discussion and their important specialized contributions: Luiz Allan Kunzle, María José Breilh; Maria Lourdes Larrea, Giannina Zamora, Bayron Torres, Mónica Izurieta; Doris Guilcamaigua, and Orlando Felicita. I thank the collaborators of the "AndinaEcoSaludable" program and the former Director of the Health Sciences Area, José Luis Coba, for their kind encouragement. In the prolonged period of this ambitious project, two other rectors of my university provided the institutional support for my work: Enrique Ayala and Cesar Montaño. I thank them sincerely. I also cherish my colleagues from other universities who during my career contributed to the development of my work, especially those at Central University of Ecuador's School of Medicine, who taught me about health and the importance of academic reform; those at the Autonomous Metropolitan University of México for providing me the knowledge and epistemological platform that made possible my first essay on critical epidemiology; those at the Collective Health Institute of the Federal University of Bahía-Brazil for giving me the means to expand my methodological and practical propositions; and those at the London School of Tropical Medicine and Hygiene for a fruitful experience to understand the power and limits of quantitative analysis.

I express very special words of gratitude to my dear friend Gerard Coffey, who laboriously made the translations from Spanish to English of some sections and the text revisions of my originals in English. I also appreciate the talented colleges and graduate students who provided key discussions and critical arguments during a variety of courses in Argentina, Bolivia, Brazil, Canada, Colombia, Costa Rica, Chile, the Dominican Republic, Ecuador, El Salvador, France, México, Peru, Portugal, the United States, and Venezuela.

Finally, I express my gratitude to all the social, community, and indigenous leaders who through their friendship and participation have made possible a productive intercultural alliance that has generated much material for this book.

ABOUT THE AUTHOR

Jaime Breilh, MD, PhD, MSc, is former Rector (President) of the Universidad Andina Simón Bolívar. He is past president of the Ecuadorian Academy of Medicine (2014–2016); coordinator of the doctoral and postdoctoral programs in "Collective Health, Environment and Society"; director of the Center for Research and Evaluation of Collective Health (CILABSalud); and creator and director of the research, graduate training, and scientific services provision program AndinaEcoSaludable). He is recognized as one of the founders of contemporary critical Latin American epidemiology (Latin American Movement of Social Medicine/ Collective Health). His numerous publications and research offer pioneering innovative contributions on research methodology, the understanding of social determination of health, critical health theory, and the history of Latin American epidemiology, with instruments for intercultural participative research.

INTRODUCTION

CRITICAL EPIDEMIOLOGY—BOLD
SCIENTIFIC THINKING AND THE
GLOBAL IRRUPTION OF INEQUITY

Critical Epidemiology and the People's Health is an act of compassionate critical intellectual pursuit and audacious resistance with which to confront an ailing world. It aims to be a valid tool for rethinking prevention and the promotion of life in a civilization that has taken inequality and social pain to their extremes. The fundamental source of its inspiration is the selfless work of many epidemiologists, physicians, nurses, professionals, scientists, and social leaders of all types and disciplines, including gender and ethnical advocates, who dedicate their lives to defend, repair, mitigate, and promote wellness and the people's health. Contemporary books won't change the present unsolicited World, but they can provide a powerful testimony of the valid contributions of premillennial generations that forged irreplaceable critical knowledge of the societies we want to transform. If millennial and postmillennial generations make good use of their particular potentialities, and free themselves of the ideological chains imposed on them in the name of youthful innovation, they will surely appreciate what good scientific work has been accomplished. If young and older conscious scholars look back at our civilization with radical wisdom, we will surely be better prepared to rescue the progressive side of the science and arts production that is synthetized in daring publications.

Today, life sciences face multifaceted global challenges that demand of us academic consistency, consciousness, and resilience. Epidemiology, as with any scientific work that is involved in the defense of well-being and health, must approach its goals with boldness and an open mind, in order to assume the knowledge and wisdom of our peoples as a vital component of research and action.

In this context, the explanatory power of science is a potent tool for social governance. It is an instrument to build and rethink the utopian goal of plentiful wellness. Be it for practical productive purposes or for political reasons, knowledge is key for social planning and evaluation. Its contribution to the interpretation and appraisal of reality has inevitably made it a tool for the construction of hegemonic or liberating ideas. This characteristic has inevitably placed scientific work under the permanent scrutiny and pressure of opposing social forces.

Sciences advance not only through an accumulation of technical knowledge. Periodically, they experience profound paradigm shifts. Physical science's reasoning and calculations, for instance, were based for many years on the seemingly immovable principles of Newtonian mechanics. Light was supposed to travel in a straight line and gravitational force was supposed to define the physical order and movement of the entire universe. But at one point the dialectic logic of relativity overturned the mechanistic dogmas and revolutionized theoretical physics. At the beginning, new ideas are rejected or made invisible by mainstream strongholds, and a process of scientific epistemicide demands creativity and resilience on the part of the reformers. As a younger discipline, epidemiology is now experiencing a paradigm shift because its previously uncontested causal linear thinking is being overturned by the dialectic principles that social determination of health theory encompasses.

Thomas Kuhn described these profound epistemological, methodological, and practical periods of transformation as a scientific revolution (Kuhn, 1970). In Chapter 3, we discuss this issue in more detail, but in these introductory reflections it will suffice to underline the fact that our discipline, as with any other scientific work dealing with the integrity of life and well-being, has developed in the historical framework of the clash of ideas and is influenced by strategic interests of socially opposed stakeholders.

It is within this contradictory and contested societal context that epidemiology, public health's so-called diagnostic arm, must operate: called on to produce objective assessments of social well-being. Both in private productive settings and in public spaces, epidemiological statements and indicators are considered to be the barometers of the health and well-being of the population. In general, these statements explicitly and implicitly evaluate the healthiness and fair-mindedness of industrial systems and of urban and rural enclaves. In doing so, they assess the effectiveness of public policy and governmental regulations. Epidemiology thereby justifies or casts doubt on companies, governmental entities, and/or the individuals and parties in power, apparently committed to the protection of human life and ecosystems.

In the 21st century, the acceleration of neoliberalism and the global monopoly of agricultural, industrial, financial, and, more recently, strategic digital resources have produced a systematic regression of human, social, and environmental rights. Globalized lobbying and corporate rule are rapidly dismantling the institutional and ethical foundations of conventional public health and environmental justice policies. Moreover, cannibalistic corporate greed has expanded unilateral control of all basic life resources and expanded social disparities (Klein, 2000). The ongoing fourth industrial revolution has spread and accelerated health inequity, enlarging unhealthy processes and landscapes.

Planetary life and human health are severely constrained by the unhealthy civilization that underlies the macroeconomic and technological apparatus, and the accelerated global decline of well-being—with hardly any substantial variation between different types of societies: those that form the largest economies in the affluent North, the emerging economies, and the rest of nations situated in the bottom of the so-called development scale—is the greatest challenge faced by responsible, grounded science.

The phenomenological expressions of this worldwide regression appear in all classes of reports. In recent decades, indicators of income inequality—a partial parameter of social inequity—have increased in nearly all world regions. In 2019, the world's billionaires, only 2,153 people, had more wealth than 4.6 billion people (Coffey et al., 2020). In 2016, the share of total national income accounted for by the powerful top 10% of the population ranged from 37% in Europe to 41% in China; 46% in Russia; 47% in the United States and Canada; approximately 55% in sub-Saharan Africa, Brazil, and India; and 61% in the Middle East (Alvaredo, Chancel, Piketty, Saez, & Zucman, 2018). The permanent rise of the wealthy inevitably leads to the constant decline of the poor (Fry & Taylor, 2018). The gap ($r > g$) between private capital rent (r) and the entire value of income and production (g) that existed throughout the 20th century is becoming even wider. This means that capital will increase more quickly than production and income. In simple terms, this regressive trend implies that the past is devouring the future (Piketty, 2015). Accumulated collective fear and anger is exploding in a wave of global protest, which gives clear expression to the continuous scientific and artistic works that have depicted the planetary regression of justice, equity, and wellness.

Paradoxically, this colossal movement revolves around the convergence of productivist uses of the technology of the fourth industrial revolution (Ribeiro, 2016); the unfair and fraudulent dispossession of strategic resources in their most varied forms (Harvey, 2003); and even the opportunistic exploitation of conditions of extreme, shock, despair, and social anxiety (Klein, 2008).

All basic means of social reproduction and the people's health are in the hands of a few corporate giants. Iron hand dominance of strategic resources and commodities is achieved through land and water grabbing (Nolte, Chamberlain, & Giger, 2016), patent-protected seed control (Kuyek, 2001), and, in general, the oligopolistic control of the food system and the imposition of a neoliberal diet (Otero, Pechlaner, Liberman, & Gürcan, 2015). The formation of huge transnational corporations stands behind the massive induction of unhealthy pro-big business consumer behaviors.

This regressive trend has been defined in the United States as "America's concentration crisis" (Open Markets Institute, 2018). It also affects a range of specific health care-related markets, from syringes to medical patient financing. A growing monopoly power in the health care sector contributes significantly to high prices, poor quality, and lack of access that millions of Americans experience when interacting with the health care system. The brilliant metaphor of "health care under the knife" clearly depicts the gravity of this corrosion of health rights (Waitzkin et al., 2018). Extreme inequality is also demolishing health rights and democracy in Latin America (Cañete et al., 2015), in the process of becoming a modern version of the old practice of bleeding and colonialism that has kept open the veins of Latin America (Galeano, 2004).

The unparalleled increase of social and health inequity is an important expression of the present worldwide breakdown of healthy life conditions. This uncontrolled growth of a technologically accelerated market economy and the intensification of neocolonial strategies in the 21st century are multiplying the threats to life on Earth.

The contemporary geographical expansion of the spaces penetrated by capital (Harvey, 2001) brings us back to the organic relationship between the modern capital reproduction and the older processes of dispossession that shaped the historical geography of capitalism from early colonial times (Harvey, 2003). Neo-extractivist structures operate through the organic interrelation of long-standing and newer mechanisms of profit extraction. On the one hand, we have the recrudescence of openly violent territorial dispossession tactics that operate through war, armed extortion by local drug lords, and even the intentional burning of rainforests to expand mining and agribusiness frontiers. These lawless procedures, combined with fraudulent financial expropriations and the cheap long-term land leasing of the most fertile soils, are simply the modern expression of the age-old dispossession of strategic natural resources. On the other hand, high-tech neo-extractivist activities in mining, agribusiness, and digital services–consumer cyber platforms—that operate with personal data as the most valued commodity—constitute its brand new face (Dance, La Forgia, & Confessore, 2018).

The curse of this new gilded age is therefore not only the *diseconomy*[1] of entrepreneurial gigantism and its structural corruptness (Wu, 2019) but also its impact on social democracy and its power to weaken the legal control of health-related behaviors and goods. This complex multidimensional regression of social and health rights explains the expansion of an array of pandemic developments or "pathologies of power" (Farmer, 2005).

The case of globalized obesity clearly illustrates the dynamic multidimensional nature of epidemiological transformation of our societies. In the broader context of big economy and political power, we find the expansion of agribusiness' obesogenic products and the corresponding corporate lobbying, which finally induced the congressional US farm bills of the 1970s. The new legal framework determined "a rapid increase in food portion sizes, accelerated marketing and affordability of energy dense foods," while at the same time inducing "widespread introduction of cheap and potent sweetening agents, such as high-fructose corn syrup, which

---

1. Scale diseconomies: To the extent that a corporation grows disproportionately, scale-up economies appear (i.e., intricate internal control system, growth of employee greed, and increasing market maladjustment). Growing power determines that as a business grows larger, it begins to enjoy different types of advantages that have less to do with the efficiency of the operation and more to do with its ability to exercise economic and political power, just or in conjunction with others.

infiltrated the food system and affected the whole population" (Rogers, Woodward, Swinburn, & Dietz, 2018). There is a clear dynamic articulation of general societal forces that subsume particular unhealthy modes of living and at the same time condition individual lifestyles and obesity as their related corporal embodiment. This constitutes an integral view in contrast with hegemonic, causal epidemiology, which interprets this global phenomenon as the generalization of an essentially personal biological or psychological problem that demands individual health care measures. Concomitantly, the unrestricted growth of pharmaceutical big business has unleashed mechanisms that distort the medical code of honor and are lethal for scientific academic control, which explains the reductionist responses that the medical establishment gives to problems such as obesity (Jones & Wilsdon, 2018).

This vertiginous, technologically based rhythm of wealth concentration places human and nature's rights in a precarious situation. The frenetic expansion of the postmodern consumerist society makes us hostages to a civilization that has imposed a new logic of living, new principles of organization, and new rhythms of life that are clearly incompatible with a healthy ethos.

Greed and its counterpart of philosophical individualism have derailed the material and spiritual fundaments of the common good that nurtured wellness and made democracy viable. Structural unfairness and extreme political shortsightedness are propelling our planet toward a true social, sanitary, environmental, and moral abyss.

However, the material mechanisms of this uncontrolled destructiveness and extremely inequitable World System are far from self-sustaining. They are clearly supported by a set of political–ideological, cultural, and communicative mechanisms that discipline collectivities and alienate them from their strategic needs. As was recently confirmed in the political crises of Brazil and Bolivia, even religious entrepreneurial ideological platforms are playing a major role in debasing social consciousness and sovereignty. New powerful multimillionaire sects subject their growing clienteles to a fundamentalist indoctrination that aims to adapt the poor people's common sense, their profound subjectivity, to the role of functional consumers and defenders of the neoliberal mode of living: a "new Christ," an inverse Christianity not of the poor but of the wealthy. In the case of Latin America, this is no longer the principal function of traditional conservative Catholicism but a new practical commercialized version of the distinct forms of imported Protestantism that assume private individual success as God's utmost reward (Arístegui, 2019). When one looks from a critical epidemiology perspective at this massive ideological alienation of impoverished urban and rural communities—both "mestizo" and ethnically indigenous and Afro—one realizes, among other things, that it implies a disdain and belligerent rejection of their original ethnic indigenous roots and cultural practices. Instead of rediscovering the wisdom of others, the richness of their health-related notions and practices, from a tolerant, knowledgeable, and democratic interculturality, and instead of sharing efforts in the intercultural search for a new civilization and healthy modes of living, fundamentalist thinking derails these constructive pathways to make racism, sexism, and intolerance the canon of social coexistence.

This is the global setback that places before the academic world the urgency of audaciously reviving critical and responsible science, as well as building a whole new intercultural participative knowledge. Health specialists therefore face the extremely complex and daunting challenge of rethinking our work from a different perspective of sensitivity, and a new paradigm.

Considering the complex and adverse scenario we have outlined, in this book we have tried to answer some important questions: What is the real challenge of critical epidemiology in an era of insatiable and cannibalistic corporate greed, bewildering deterioration of the planet's natural reserves, and imposition of colonizing and patriarchal devastating societal canons? What should be the guiding questions in all responsible and sensitive research centers and academic scenarios? What, then, is a rigorous, updated, and effective epidemiology? What is its role in the face of our most urgent needs, both in the Global North and in the Global South?

It has been argued for a long time that consistent advances in epidemiological method are centrally related to the sophistication of induction (i.e., reliability and validity) and statistical models (Miettinen, 1985) and sophistication of data management. All this in order to better describe risk factors and predict focalized outcomes. More recently, mainstream conventional researchers concerned with the changing nature of present conceptions and practices denote a growing acceptance of the "scientificity" of qualitative research. Either to enhance the traditional method or as a complementary and equally valid tool, so-called interpretative research holds a new position in the academic world. This obeys the need to recognize new ways for addressing new kinds of questions, shifting the balance between the researcher and the researched, and adding conceptual and theoretical depth to knowledge (Popay, 2003).

The book will deal with this quantitative versus qualitative debate, and other complementary issues—an important but essentially instrumental discussion—but its cognitive and strategic purpose is to go beyond instrumental discussion, to delineate a different epistemological and hands-on perspective: a historically defined standpoint for transformative action in the face of ever growing health needs of our time.

The history of all fields of science demonstrates that the contents and guiding strategies of its intellectual and practical operations change permanently. In his magnificent book *Revolution in Science*, I. Cohen (1985) reveals cornerstone arguments about the changing nature of scientific work. For the purpose of this introduction, I summarize his fundamental explanations of the profound changes that interpretative models, values, and social connections of science experience in different societies and historical periods. In his opinion, those new routes are determined by the use of the evolving ideas of each period; the creative application of ideas of other disciplines; the two-way interaction between the natural and exact sciences and the social and behavioral sciences; and, most important, the fact that revolutionary moves in science are not produced by instrumental innovation (i.e., quantitative or qualitative) but by the application of a groundbreaking theory or set of revolutionary ideas[2]—a paradigm in Kuhn's terms (Kuhn, 1962).

So, when analyzing the development of any scientific tradition, we must recognize that beyond the sociopolitical frame, the

---

2. Cohen from his rationalistic perspective illustrates this with the case of Galileo's revolution in astronomy: "Astronomy was never the same again. But these revolutionary

development of powerful ideas that spring out of needs, especially at crucial times, does inspire and guide transcendent, renewing, academic work.

In this introduction to *Critical Epidemiology and the People's Health*, it is important to highlight some of those instigating thoughts that have recurrently influenced the construction of the Latin American critical epidemiology paradigm. The book constitutes our first complete and wide-ranging English account of the theoretical and practical elements of our proposal for a critical epidemiology; until this time I have only published complete books and work of this scale regarding my version of the Latin American paradigm, in Spanish and Portuguese.

The first and probably the most significant intellectual challenge responds to the need to re-examine, and overturn, the governing epistemological and ethical canons of the mainstream health sciences, in the process, repositioning the cardinal importance of critical science. This implies providing a convincing critique of the supposed pillars of the supposedly rigorous conventional Cartesian paradigms of hegemonic thinking. In all times, this dialectical move has always proved vital to protect academic knowledge from economic and political co-optation. Currently, the paramount importance of a critical epistemology therefore

---

changes (including the visual demonstrations the Ptolemaic system is false) were not 'produced' by the telescope but by Galileo's theoretical ideas drawing Copernican and unorthodox conclusions from his telescopic observations. The telescope produced a vast change in kind, magnitude and scope of the data base of astronomy, providing the observational materials on which revolution would eventually become founded; but these data did not in and of themselves constitute a revolution in science" (p. 9).

relates to the urgent need to protect and refresh the traditions of independent, responsible, critical health science.

In the second place, given the present affliction of our societies—both in the Global South and in the Global North—what is at stake is also the condemnation and questioning of a permissive or sometimes even mercenary epidemiology that, whether we like it or not, has become an accomplice of the historical hegemonic project. We must consequently embrace and increase with all our talent and ethical reserves the emancipatory force of the critical epidemiological paradigm, in order to denounce and counteract a decadent civilization and its grasping and shortsighted economic system.

Radical science has flourished in long-term intellectual traditions both in the South and in the North. A personal anecdote will serve at this point to illustrate their complementary nature. Two years ago, I was conducting a seminar discussion with my doctoral students about the construction of a transdisciplinary intercultural critique of the eco-epidemiological consequences of agribusiness. That activity coincided with an invitation to speak at the American Public Health Association annual meeting (APHA 2017) in its Spirit of 1848 Caucus Section. I gladly accepted the honor of joining a representative group of top-notch North American critical scholars and presenting my theory on "the 4 S's of life and the Andean academic-people's epidemiological approach." Inevitably I had to study the guiding principles of the Spirit of 1848 APHA caucus and understand its complementarity with our Latin American collective health movement philosophy. On doing so, my attention was drawn to Rudolph Virchow's sobering argument: "Preserving health and preventing

disease requires 'full and unlimited democracy' and radical measures rather than 'mere palliatives' " (Virchow, 1848). Going over
Virchow's powerful statement, I recalled the pioneering epidemiological writings of Eugenio Espejo—not only one of the forefathers
of Latin American Independence but also a medical revolutionary
from Quito—who authored a groundbreaking volume on his
socio-epidemiological argument relating smallpox with health
inequity and criticizing a dominant bureaucracy (Espejo, 1785/
1994). The radical pioneering ideas contained in Espejo's essay,
written in Spanish and published in Madrid, soon crossed the colonial frontiers of the "Royal Audiencia of Quito" and his innovative arguments were expeditiously translated to Italian (1789)
and German (1795), as explained by the medical historian Nuñez
(2018).

This conceptual parallelism of critical voices coming from distinct settings both in the South and in the North of America is by
no means a minor coincidence. It exemplifies the epistemological
identity of bodies of knowledge linked to emancipatory science.

My dear colleague Nancy Krieger, of the prestigious Department
of Social and Behavioral Sciences of the Harvard T.H. Chan School
of Public Health, kindly invited me to present in this contribution to the "Small Book Big Ideas" series that she proposed, for the
first time in the English language a complete synthesis of all the
cardinal elements of my new epidemiology proposition; not with-
standing some abridged previous publications focusing on certain
facets of work. I immediately accepted, considering it an unparalleled personal opportunity to contribute to international socially
supportive academic work. I was especially encouraged by her design of the series. An important motivation for my enthusiasm was

also the fact that the series is being produced in partnership with Oxford University Press (OUP), a prominent, well-renowned scientific publisher. Chad Zimmerman, former Clinical Medicine Editor of OUP, suggested that in this small book I provide a consistent panorama of my own ideas and contributions to Latin American epidemiology.

The significant undertaking of translating for an English-speaking audience my key ideas about the nature and responsibilities of epidemiological research implies a double challenge. First is the need to overcome a cultural barrier. In effect, despite the fact that many of my epidemiological works have received wide circulation in Spanish and Portuguese in prestigious doctoral and postdoctoral programs of the region, and although many of them have also been defined as cutting-edge contributions by leading North American health scientists (Briggs, 2005; Krieger, 2011; Waitzkin, Iriart, Estrada, & Lamadrid, 2001), to date they have not been widely disseminated in the English-speaking world. Second, and most important, it implies the complex challenge of polishing and communicating a well-knit synthesis of my principal contributions by placing my ideas within the logic, framework, and structure of English academic writing. In accepting this challenge, I have been encouraged by the very positive experience of postgraduate lecturing at the University of California (UC). Professor Charles Briggs, a leading internationally known social scientist and knowledgeable expert on Latin America, invited me to lecture in a full quarter program of undergraduate and graduate studies at UC San Diego and, more recently, a doctoral seminar at Berkeley. Both were proposed by the respective Latin American Studies Centers of the UC branch and, in the second case, sponsored by the prestigious National Nurses United and the California Nurses Association.

I sincerely hope that this collaborative effort will open a path to consistent intercultural cooperation and mutual intellectual enquiry. The book is intended, on the conceptual side, to present our efforts in rethinking the scope of wellness and healthy living in a contextualized manner. It also presents an alternative logic for constructing the real object, subject, and practical projection of transformative health knowledge: a counteractive trend involving concrete methodological restatements needed for complex thinking in epidemiology. That is, complex, intercultural, and emancipating knowledge–wisdom research that involves, but also supersedes, the innovation of formal quantitative models.

In other words, critical epidemiology must avoid juxtaposing a critical model of relationships within society and the practices needed to change it, with the passive, functional, value-free conventional cognitive structure of empirical analysis. It must be consistent with a renewed methodological perspective that breaks away from the Cartesian rigidities of a positivistic notion of correspondence and objectivity. This means it must override the *active object—passive subject* unidirectional reflex conception of empirical method and, at the same time, supersede the *active subject—passive object* logic of cultural relativism. It must therefore acquire an *active object—active subject* form of logic that can only be fully developed in the context of *active epidemiological praxis*. All three elements must therefore be considered and operated as active interdependent elements of the movement of emancipatory knowledge needed to explain, mobilize, and transform society, and not merely describe its fragmented causal conjunctions.

The previous reasoning leads to a discussion of what is hard social science or, specifically, hard epidemiology. The "hardness" of epidemiology does not only reside in rigorous objectivity but also simultaneously resides in a laborious and well-knit subjectivity, and also an effective integration of praxis. What we need is a triangular action that articulates three fundamental elements: (1) a solid transformative project of the critical processes involved in the social determination of a certain epidemiological condition; (2) a clearly integrated block of affected or concerned collectivities; and (3) a solid and effective integration of intercultural, transdisciplinary, transformative knowledge in action. Integral, intercultural, meta-critic epidemiological method needs this triple movement to mobilize society toward the prevention of unhealthy processes and promotion of protective modes of living, at all levels of the social determination of health movement.

One challenge of this book is to show how we have gone about rethinking the *object–subject–praxis movement*. This is crucial in defining sharp theoretical, technical, social, and administrative ways to act in defense of life and enhance healthy modes of living. In order to attain that objective, we need to unravel the incomplete and compliant logic and structure of empiricist science. It is our ethical duty to overcome the paramount rule of the causal epidemiological method in bureaucratic planning and functionalist research. We must elucidate a means of recovering the dialectic inductive–deductive–praxis movement, where the construction of study object and study subject become interdependent and define its movement in the context of transformative social praxis.

This brief book summarizes our work and our main propositions—stated in many previous books and articles—constructed in the mainstream of the Latin American social medicine/collective health movement. It also incorporates the reflections and clarifications that appeared while condensing that experience for an English-speaking public.

The guiding principle of my work has been, for many years now, the need to promote and consolidate effective intercultural research in the intersection of academic and progressive community paradigm building. We still are far from completing the task, but we already have some very powerful and interesting successes.

In Chapter 1, I present a panoramic analysis of the roots and landmarks of the critical scientific tradition: the new philosophy and ethics of the Latin American critical collective health sciences. When streamlining our initial essay text, we came to understand that it was important to start by familiarizing our readers with our work and its historical construction.

In Chapter 2, I deal with the global problems that make critical epidemiology an imperative tool in our current world. It aims to explain my epidemiological understanding of the historically demanding socio-environmental contradictions, out of which we must extract the critical processes that must be central to our work. I emphasize the fact that greedy destructive big business applications of new technologies of the fourth industrial revolution have left planetary life and health hanging by a thread; they are the basis of a civilization in which producing fast, living fast, and dying fast is the logic and foundation of accelerated profit. We stress the need to expose the fast-track, unhealthy, global civilization of the 21st century and to redefine the scope of wellness and health.

Chapter 3 describes the main conceptual and methodological breaks and new categories that I have proposed in order to go beyond the Cartesian logic. Basically, I have condensed this movement into five central ruptures with the cognitive pillars of empirical epidemiology: lineal causality, external conjunction, empirical quantitative and qualitative analysis, empirical socio-epidemiological stratification, and Cartesian health geography. To illustrate my reasoning, I have inserted some examples taken from our research and postgraduate teaching.

Chapter 3 also highlights some key elements for working toward a new framework for practice and ethos, one necessary to subvert the notions of health prevention and promotion and to move from passive vertical bureaucratic surveillance to an active, community-based critical health monitoring movement. Here, the overall intention is to move our reasoning away from functionalist public health to incorporate the transformative notion of collective health. This is a complex operation that presupposes the need to move beyond conventional conceptions, to leave our institutional comfort zones, to reaffirm a critical scientific philosophy, and to rescue potent concepts of the wisdom of "others."

The final question we need to answer in this introduction is: Who is this book for? We have made an effort to incorporate in this synthesis of our work a basic streamlined version of key theoretical and methodological elements that the reader can expand through our bibliography. The book is intended for curious, up-to-date, open-minded, and, above all, aware physicians, health professionals, social scientists, social leaders, health and social workers, gender and health rights advocates, and community leaders. People who are willing to distance themselves from the dominant health paradigm, as well as teachers who are willing to inspire their students to leave their academic and professional comfort zones in order to restate their relationship to people.

In his handwritten letter to Robert Markus (February 1950), Albert Einstein wrote:

> A human being is a part of the whole called by us universe, a part limited in time and space. He experiences himself, his thoughts and feelings as something separated from the rest. . . . Our task must be to free ourselves . . . by widening our circle of compassion to embrace all living creatures and the whole of nature in its beauty.

I sincerely hope that after reading this book about the pressing epidemiological challenges and ethical duties we face in our present civilization, readers will warmly endorse his wise invitation to assume the protection of human and natural life, and will accept it as the leitmotiv of epidemiology.

LATIN AMERICAN CRITICAL EPIDEMIOLOGY

THE ROOTS AND LANDMARKS OF A SCIENTIFIC TRADITION

The scientific traditions present in the field of epidemiology have varied at different times and places according to their theoretical–methodological fundamentals, their symbolic elements, and their social commitments/values. In order to understand a scientific tradition, one must identify its central characterizing paradigm.[1] Researchers, teachers, specialists, and intellectuals are commonly grouped around paradigms that define their views, priorities, and practical strategies.

In previous work, I have discussed an innovative view of Kuhn's (1962) theory in order to demonstrate, from a broader sociological perspective, the important role that paradigms played in the different traditions and "schools" of epidemiology and, above all, to explain why the history of our discipline shows periodic interpretative and political clashes (Figure 1.1; Breilh, 2003a).

---

1. The concept *paradigm* was coined by Thomas Kuhn (1962) to define a consistent structure or disciplinary matrix (symbolic generalizations, beliefs, values, models, and network of concepts) through which scientists view their field; also implying the theoretical–methodological beliefs that define problematic options, methods, and commitments.

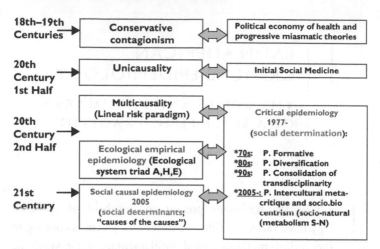

Figure 1.1 Epidemiological paradigm clash in Latin American history.

Adapted from Breilh, J. (2003). *Epidemiología crítica ciencia emancipadora e inter-culturalidad*. Buenos Aires, Argentina: Lugar Editorial. This 7th edition comes from an initial thesis dissertation of 1977-Autonomous University of Xochimilco that circu-lated as such and then in 1979 the first edition was published in Quito, Ecuador by Universidad Central.

Opposing perspectives and methodological differences arise in all periods, representing the interests and views of scholars and decision-makers that adhere to different philosophical and prac-tical postures, which are encompassed by opposing logics related to the origin and management of health problems. Epidemiology is no exception to the historically contested development of academic work. Some key historical controversies can be highlighted: the clash of conservative *contagionism* with the more progressive *political economy* and miasmatic doctrines in the 19th century; the confrontation between unicausal explanations and the foundational groundbreaking works of social medicine in the first half of the 20th century; and, in later times, the opposition of both the functionalist linear multicausal and the ecological empirical epidemiology paradigms—together with their operational arm, the risk paradigm—with different versions of critical epidemiology from the second half of the 20th century to the present day (Almeida, 2000; Breilh, 2003a, 2015a; Tesh, 1988).

What is relevant at this point is to understand that epidemiology has moved through time under specific conditions and pressures that have contributed to its conceptual and practical shape. This occurs because scientific knowledge is socially determined. Contextual power relations intervene through economic, institutional, and cultural mediations that condition the material–financial, symbolic, and ideological settings of research. But they also determine the modes of living and social relations of researchers. Their vocations, values, preferences, technical appeals, and resources, as well as the dynamics of their concrete acts of creation, are socially shaped. With time, this process of socially determined activities is embodied in concrete interpretative models and research designs.

As public health's so-called diagnostic arm, epidemiology operates under great social pressure. The different interpretations of social development, assessments of well-being, and conceptions of health confront scientists and decision-makers situated on opposite ends of the political spectrum. Epidemiological statements and indicators are assumed to be valuable measurements of the population's health and well-being. Those statements explicitly and implicitly provide an image of the effectiveness of the institutional and economic entities responsible for producing a variety of health actions, of their public policies, and of individual decision-makers in governing positions.

Emblematic Representatives of the Latin American Critical Health Science Tradition

The construction of contemporary Latin American critical conceptions about epidemiology can be viewed from different perspectives and emphases. In this section, we discuss characterizing events and names from the American South in order to profile basic contributions and origins. We also briefly note the fundamental influence of personalities from the North that are clearly linked to the development of our critical ideas.

The social medicine/collective health movement's construction of a renewed perspective of the health sciences drew its lever knowledge and inspiring practices from three fundamental sources, allowing for a cumulative process that was rebuilt in the early 20th century and has grown continuously to the present day: (1) the enlightening academic health studies centered on the transformation of functionalist public health paradigms; (2) the powerful contributions of feminism and gender-related health; and (3) more recently, the influence of the philosophical and cultural critique of the indigenous people's movement.

The *Latin American critical social medicine tradition* can be traced back to colonial times. The 16th-century colonial system fractured the communitarian spirit of the indigenous societies. A complex class and cast system of inequitable colonial relations replaced the indigenous people's notion of a communal, social organization based on solidarity. The colonial state organized blood and fire governance and imposed, by means of inquisitorial force, the marginalization of peasants and urban poor. The colonial regime institutionalized not only social exclusion but also white supremacist unicultural thinking, racism, and sexism (ethnic and gender epistemicide). In that context, not only was the pre-colonial egalitarian ethos broken but also the harmonious conception and management of Nature of our native societies was shattered.

In colonial society, the violent expropriation of gold and land and the feudal exploitation of the labor force in agricultural fiefs and mines formed the basis of society. However, the golden rule was not only greed and the concentration of material goods but also political and cultural subordination. Cultural unilateral dominance and *epistemicide*[2] resulted in a loss of many forms of sophisticated native knowledge, including the health knowledge of the time.

As has been the case in many repressive societal periods, emancipatory thought flourished in the colonial era. The need for emancipating ideas explains the libertarian nature of the works of Eugenio Espejo, a physician, writer, and journalist who was an outstanding and inspiring figure during the period preceding the anti-colonial struggle. It also accounts for his virtuous, pioneering concepts on social determination of health. Together with his sister Manuela—another enlightened combatant—and José Mejía Lequerica, a notable reformer, Espejo not only inspired the

---

2. Epistemicide refers to the killing of a knowledge system.

Latin American libertarian struggle of the 18th century but also provided groundbreaking contributions, both as a writer and as a medical scientist, that headed the construction of a new paradigm for various fields of knowledge, including epidemiology (Breilh, 2001, 2016).

The importance of Espejo transcends the national scientific and epistemological spectrum. In some of my previous publications, I insisted on the need to revisit Espejo's multifaceted contributions to the history of the health sciences. For many years, his biographers have been trapped in a reductionist biomedical appraisal of his work. But in order to understand his essential contributions to epidemiology, it is necessary to go beyond his clinical–therapeutic endeavors and capture his original contributions that help explain health as a socially determined phenomenon. To oppose the theocratic foundations of scholastic medicine, the founder of Ecuadorian critical epidemiology was obliged to work within the paradigm of Enlightened humanism. It was his thirst for justice that impelled Espejo to build a multi-dimensional critique of colonial society and its economic, social, cultural, and political foundations. One can only grasp the essence of his comprehensive critical revolutionary ideas by locating them within an integral emancipatory project. In doing so, the articulation of his conceptions of health as part of a coherent anti-colonial system of thought can be clearly seen.

For the purpose of the current analysis, we highlight Espejo's groundbreaking *Reflections on a Safe Method to Protect the People from Smallpox* (1994), in which he lays out his socio-epidemiological argument relating smallpox to health inequity and criticizing a dominant bureaucracy. The radical, pioneering ideas contained in Espejo's essay were originally written in Spanish and published in Madrid, but they soon crossed the colonial frontiers of the Royal Audiencia of Quito, and his innovative arguments were expeditiously translated to Italian (1789) and German (1795), as explained by the medical historian Nuñez (2018).

Thus, in his *Reflections* (1785/1994), rather than a replica on the treatment and specific measures of prevention of smallpox, Espejo offers to the history of science a consistent evaluation of the prevailing European ideas of his time, inserting the explanation of the disease and its transmission into the logic of social determination of malady. He assumed the "anti-contagionist" thesis from a visionary perspective—a position that was only defined as revolutionary in Europe a century later. To do so, he questioned the method of Spanish specialist Don Francisco Gil, whose explanation relied on supposedly "external" or foreign contagions that would introduce the disease from the outside. On the contrary, Espejo proclaimed that the "internal" ways of living of colonial society were to be blamed. He stated,

> The landowner is making his fortune at the cost of the misery and hunger of the public and the indolence of the usurers, of the merchants, and the cruel greed of the producers who hide wheat to sell it at a higher price, setting then his wealth in the hunger and agony of the poor. (p. 77)

Espejo was a pioneer of a critical scientific tradition of health and wellness. While revealing the limits of 18th-century knowledge, his works constitute a foundational milestone of renewed thought in the health sciences and most likely in the sciences in general. His brilliant comprehensive criticism of colonial society has been defined as a cornerstone for restating the origins of libertarian Latin American philosophy (Roig, 2013). Espejo created an epistemological democratizing umbrella of emancipatory scientific ideas on health and society that, in the case of Ecuadorian medicine, was reclaimed 150 years later when the social medicine thinkers confronted the country's oligarchic and class-based society during the so-called Julian Revolution period of the early 20th century. A turning point towards social and health and cultural rights were two scientists Isidro Ayora—medical doctor and reformist that lead the State's transformation as president—and Luís Telmo Paz y Miño—military leader, geographer, demographer, linguist and writer-, played key political roles in this transformative period.

The pillars of modern so-called Western social medicine that influenced the development of public health and epidemiology are found in innovative contributions from both the North and the South during the 19th century and the first half of the 20th century. In effect, this powerful European tradition dates back to revolutionary works of 19th-century thinkers. One outstanding representative is Rudolf Virchow (Germany), with his emblematic and inspiring call for action, inscribed in his report of a typhus epidemic, in which he clearly stated that "preserving health and preventing disease requires 'full and unlimited democracy' and radical measures rather than 'mere palliatives'" (Espejo, 1930; Virchow, 1848). Henry Sigerist (France) expanded the horizon of critical health sciences with his potent *Civilization and Disease* (1945), which made an outspoken pioneering contribution to the broadening of health science by incorporating the role of economics, culture, philosophy, the arts, and an interdisciplinary approach to the understanding of health. George Rosen's *History of Public Health* (1958) made crucial contributions to the progressive understanding of the origins, historical transformations, and socially determined conditions of public health. These authors' works inspired the many workshops on the critique of functionalist public health that have been held in Latin America since the 1970s.

In the mid-20th century, the work of Salvador Allende (1939) shone in South America. Allende's report, "On the Chilean Sociomedical Reality," recognized the relationship between political economy, disease, and suffering by focusing its "causal" gaze on the role of empire, underdevelopment, and the need for structural change in the life of the proletarian classes as the fundamental solution to health inequality (Waitzkin, 2011). That is, this second source of critical epidemiology did not derive solely from the works of 19th-century Europeans but, rather, had other pivotal proponents in Latin America whose contributions, often silenced by official history, must be rescued.

In effect, as a result of the turbulence and social awareness of the early decades of the past century, there was a consolidation of revolutionary social ideas that penetrated thought about health and health inequalities. This consolidation favored the emergence of other figures dedicated to critical thinking about epidemiology, such as Ricardo Paredes (1938), who, as a physician, rigorously studied the social, workplace, and health conditions of the workers of a mining company. Paredes later published a remarkable and pioneering epidemiological essay on the determination of health in early multinational mega-mining. The essay, supported by robust sociological thought and statistical evidence, provided a profound analysis of the destruction of health and the environment in Ecuador (Paredes, 1938). The works of Ramón Carrillo (1951) are also fundamental to the consolidation of this perspective. These include the *Synthetic Public Health Plan for Argentina*, in which Carrillo situates epidemiological thought as central to the search for equity and the creation of a profound vision of disease prevention.

The previously mentioned works, as Howard Waitzkin argues in his magnificent critique of medicine and public health in *Medicine and Public Health at the End of Empire* (2011), created a new perspective of social medicine and documented the impact of early capitalism.

Development of the Contemporary Latin American Social Medicine (Collective Health) Movement: 1975–2019

Cardinal Concepts: Collective Health

In order to fully understand the historical development of social medicine/collective health from a critical epistemological perspective, it is necessary to interweave the sequence of social transformations with the important academic changes that occurred during different periods. Because concepts are essential for the understanding of academic advance, we preface this section with a clarifying summary of key categories.

The concept *collective health* was coined in Latin America in 1979 and linked to the sanitary reform movement in Brazil (Nunes, 1996). Retaking ideas expressed in multiple congresses and seminars, this concept was proposed in order to overcome the dominant biomedical and conventional public health paradigms. The need was to create an explicit conceptual and practical differentiation between collective health and two other related notions: individual health and public health (Figure 1.2).

Individual health involves personal phenomena that are observed, explained, cared for, or confronted at the level of familiar everyday life. It is aimed at determining individual health patterns, exposures, and vulnerabilities and their relation to daily styles of living with their individual expressions of wellness, illness, and health needs and satisfaction. On the other hand, *public health* pertains to the institutional duties of public services for populations that are covered according to norms and regulations. It constitutes an important sphere of action, but it does not account for many other forms and areas of action that exceed those formal responsibilities covered by official or private–social

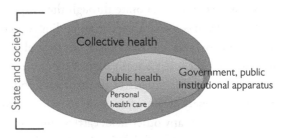

Figure 1.2 Collective, public, and individual health.

entities. Collective health involves social community-based phenomena that are produced, observed, and confronted in society. It therefore is concerned with collectively organized action centered on integrated socially based processes, either to prevent their destructive and promote their favorable health aspects or to secure reparation of harm to natural or human life.

In all three domains, health is a polysemic category. First, we need to define health as a multidimensional concrete object, considering its existence not as a theory of being but, rather, related to the direct materiality of tangible life and its cultural expressions (Lukács, 2013). This ontological dimension of health encompasses both concrete healthy, life-supportive, protecting processes and, conversely, concrete unhealthy, harmful, and destructive processes that develop in the general (societal), particular (group), and individual (phenotype, genotype, mind, and spiritual) dimensions. In Chapter 3, we expand on this important matter and the categories needed to understand those dimensions. Second, health is a *subjective construction* that springs from strategic needs of distinct groups, formed around their class position, intertwined with gender and ethnic sociocultural relations. The subjective health domain consists of a set of ideas that collective subjects must elaborate through their experience in order to understand and cope with the corresponding consequences of social determination and reproduction. Knowledgeable empowerment and control over science form part of the power relations of society needed to master subjective constructions about health and counter the dominant misinterpretations. In this regard, scientific work in health, as in any other field, carries inherent symbolic components and is thus "a transformed, subordinated, transmuted, and sometimes unrecognizable expression of the power relations of a society" (Bourdieu, 1998, p. 77). In our analysis, those relations involve the imposition of a system of social dominance and of the mistreatment of nature, forming part of a system that materially reproduces unsustainable, inequitable, and unhealthy societies and ecosystem relations, at the same time imposing a conceptual framework that justifies them. Finally, the positive transformation of concrete health conditions and the ideas involved in that transformation occur in a defined *field of action* or praxis. The practical grounds, experiences, and relations that form part of any scientific endeavor constitute the real driving and directional force of a field of discipline. These three interdependent aspects of health merit an integral multidimensional understanding (Figure 1.3).

The historic struggle for the development of *collective health* required the confluence of a determined social space, the existence of an active social block of concerned and affected collectivities, and the technical skills to apply a socially defined agenda in the

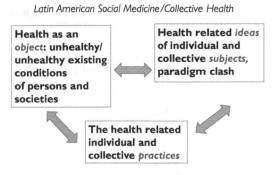

Latin American Social Medicine/Collective Health

Health as an *object*: unhealthy/ unhealthy existing conditions of persons and societies

Health related *ideas* of individual and collective *subjects*, paradigm clash

The health related individual and collective *practices*

Figure 1.3 Health as complex polysemic concept.

Breilh, J. (2003). *Epidemiología crítica ciencia emancipadora e interculturalidad* (2nd ed.). Buenos Aires, Argentina: Lugar Editorial; and Breilh, J. (2016). *Espejo adelantado de la ciencia crítica (una "antihistoria" de sus ideas en salud)*. Quito, Ecuador: Universidad Andina Simón Bolívar y Corporación Editora Nacional.

struggle for health equity and integral social transformation toward a healthy society.

The Construction of Contemporary Latin American Social Medicine/Collective Health

The interpretative models of science are a product of a complex process of the social determination of knowledge. In different historical periods, epistemic relations are built on the interpretative models that scientists develop, conventional knowledge matrices [paradigms in the Kuhnian sense (Kuhn, 1962)], and the sociopolitical–cultural conditions of broader society. These elements interweave dynamically in determining the transformation of contents, values, social compromises, directions, and practical applications of knowledge (Figure 1.4; Breilh, 2003a).

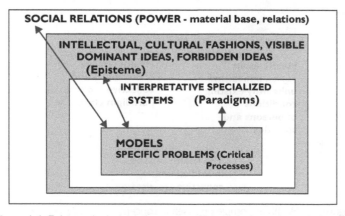

Figure 1.4 Epistemological relations: scientific knowledge, culture, and social (power) relations.

Breilh, J. (2003). *Epidemiología crítica ciencia emancipadora e interculturalidad* (2nd ed.). Buenos Aires, Argentina: Lugar Editorial.

In the Latin American "South," the extreme political authoritarianism and social inequity of the early 20th century impelled and inspired a culture of critique and resilience within the region, leaving a deep impression on social and health scientists. The growing unfairness of the broader world economy and permanent reproduction of colonialist academic relations also triggered the urge for sovereign, independent academic thinking.

Brief Periodization of the Critical Social Medicine/Collective Health Movement: Scenarios, Study Objects, and Stakeholders

In previous work, we proposed a periodization of Latin American social medicine's development: its historic settings, cardinal debates, and the stakeholders involved (Breilh, 2010, 2003a, 2016). Motivated by the need to contextualize our analysis of the epistemological framework of epidemiological development, we defined consistent relations between periods.

In doing so, important bibliographical studies have been invaluable: the vast contribution of Everardo Duarte Nunes, *Social Sciences and Health in Latin America* (1986); the review of *Debates in Social Medicine* (Franco, Nunes, Breilh, & Laurell, 1991); the brilliant updated periodization of Ana Lucia Casallas (2019); and the formidable compilation and digital library on Latin American social medicine inspired by Howard Waitzkin (University of New Mexico; https://digitalrepository.unm.edu/lasm).

The Latin American social medicine movement was founded in 1984 during the Third Latin American Seminar on Social Medicine (Ouro Preto, Brazil). Its founding was a result of a decade-long process that began in the 1970s as a reaction to a prolonged history of regional health inequity. Scholars, researchers, social leaders, and students converged from countries in which powerful nuclei had been built. Conditions were apt and the time was ripe to institutionalize the annual meetings that representative academic and social groups and organizations had been holding since the mid-1970s. The transformation of the historic social scenarios facilitated the appearance of different periods of social medicine.

Combining the historic features, social agendas, disciplinary arrangements, and epistemological ruptures that were present at different moments, four main periods in the development of Latin American social medicine can be recognized: (1) formative, initial ruptures (1970s); (2) diversification—transformative knowledge (object and subject), instrumental progress, and institutional-ization (1980s); (3) the consolidation of transdisciplinarity and initial interculturality (1990s); and (4) the consolidation of an intercultural meta-critique[3] and social–biocentric models (social–natural metabolism) (Table 1.1).

The formative period (1970s) entailed significant initial ruptures with the biomedical and conventional public health paradigms. These took place in the context of industrialism and the formal recognition of economic and social rights. In those years, social demands were basically constructed around the historical agreement or social pact between companies and formal workers. Nevertheless, during the same time period, the rise of subsalaried hiring changed labor relations in the countryside. Peripheral so-cial formations in the South constituted scenarios of imperfect

---

3. Meta-critique, which is discussed in Chapter 3, refers to the convergence of diverse critical epistemologies to explain the dominant system of social reproduction and its civilization.

Table 1.1 Periods of Latin American Social Medicine/Collective Health

Period	Characteristic Features	Agenda
Formative, initial ruptures: 1970s	Industrialism, worker and subproletarian growth Social pact for baseline rights Consolidation of primary export economy, social inequality	Rupture against pharma-biomedical model Initial deconstruction of positivism and empirical methodology Works on class analysis Initial critique of functionalist behaviorist social sciences First social medicine postgraduate programs
Diversification: transformative knowledge (object and subject) instrumental progress and institutionalization: 1980s	Neoliberalism: takeoff of extractivist productivism Aggressive privatization of health and life goods Appearance of nonproletarian social subjects: gender, ethnicity	Struggle against neoliberal anti-state policies and privatization Founding works on gender and ethnicity Gender and ethnocultural components in postgraduate programs
Consolidation of ransdisciplinarity and initial interculturality: 1990s	Initial crisis of hegemony of aggressive productivism "Progressive" extractivism, redistributive governance (neoproductivism)	Generalized ethnic, gender, and urban social movements Consolidation of critical interculturality; dialogue of knowledge—academic and popular—and practices in collective health

(continued)

Table 1.1 Continued

Period	Characteristic Features	Agenda
		Constituent projects, new constitution, and legal reformAdvancements in health system reform (two tracks): Unified health system and expansion of public social insurance Conduction of important universities, high government positions
Consolidation of an intercultural meta-critique and social–biocentrism (social–natural metabolism): 2017–	Global acceleration of capital accumulation (New information and communication technologies fourth industrial revolution—convergence, dispossession, and shock); postwork; cyber determination; artificial intelligence algorithms governance Irruption of global multiple environmental crisis and extreme climate warming; Global social protest	Demand for new civilization: 4 "S's" and Sumak Kawsay (struggle against extractivism) Religious fundamentalist entrepreneurial offensive against a new civilization Pluricultural democracy Reframing regional integration Reframing constitutional and health rights in the face of social determination of health Transdisciplinary, intercultural emancipatory knowledge Methodological theoretical construction of social metacriticism

Breilh, J. (2003a). Epidemiología crítica ciencia emancipadora e interculturalidad. Buenos Aires, Argentina: Lugar Editorial; and Breilh, J. (2013). Ciencia crítica por la vida en tiempos de una sociedad de la muerte. Divulgação em Saúde Para Debate: Centro Brasileiro de Estudos de Saúde, 49, 10–14.

dependent capitalist development. The social agenda highlighted the demands of the working class and subsalaried workers in the countryside, who ceased to be a reserve army and became an irregular mass of subsalaried workers. The social demands of the period were correspondingly focused on the responsibility of the state to provide access to rights and to democratize public services such as health and education. Social medicine had to break the mold of closed-door, curative medical care settings sustained by the emerging pharmaceutical and health care industries of the South. Mainstream medicine was impermeable to the social reality that generated the problems that arose in offices and hospitals. It was essential to break the biomedical paradigm, overcoming the idea of "health as an absence of disease," or even the supposedly broader World Health Organization (WHO) definition that conceptualizes health as the "complete physical, mental and social well-being, and not just the absence of disease."[4] These conceptualizations have not allowed health to be understood as a complex, multidimensional process but, rather, just as individual or psycho-perceptual and reduced to the narrow limits of disorders and perception of the degree of individual well-being. The incongruity of the pharmacobiomedical paradigm had to be investigated and denounced. At that time, this critique confronted a generalized uncontested biomedical dominance. It was a visionary outlook that declared a crucial counteractive movement. Today, it has been reaffirmed not only in the magnificent research

---

4. As conceptualized by WHO in a declaration approved during the International Health Conference of 1946, applied on April 7, 1948 (http://apps.who.int/gb/bd/PDF/bd47/SP/constitucion-sp.pdf).

of social medicine specialists such as Waitzkin and many others but also in the recent coherent analyses of "insiders" who meticulously uncover the flaws of mainstream medical research. This critique is based on a penetrating inventory of what two distinguished Royal Society (United Kingdom) scientists have described as the "biomedical bubble" (Jones & Wilsdon, 2018). Due to its biased priorities, lack of diversity, and systematic waste of financial resources, the model has been described as an overvalued waste. Underlying its historically earned prestige, they explain how it has become a speculative fraud that overestimates the effect of certain drugs and rules out investment in and academic concern about the real health problems of society. At the same time, corporate influence also puts pressure on public health entities, their scope of concern, and their mandate.

In this formative phase, many of us in progressive universities and research centers began to work on the broader health-related contradictions of society. We applied the potent critical arsenal of critical realism, political economy, and the serious contributions of ecology, sociology, and biology. In those initial, still immature academic endeavors, some groundbreaking conceptual and methodological arguments were profiled. We turned them into the publications of those who later formed the Latin American Latin American Social Medicine Association. At that time, some important research dealt with the relationship between productive forms, social class, and health; the productive system and working conditions as fundamental categories to reveal the intimate link between the social and the biological; and the first theoretical approximations regarding the cardinal problems of the state— health practice and education.

The historic meetings of Cuenca I (Ecuador, 1972) and Cuenca II (Ecuador, 1974), organized under the guidance of Juan Cesar García (a notable thinker of social medicine in those years), our founding group elaborated the first formal critique of the positivist conception of public health and the class-based organization of the state and health governance. New categories were embraced in the proposal for a new pathway for the movement's development. It was a time of multiple ruptures with the empirical constructions of the old public health paradigm: the positivist, lineal, causal paradigm that constrained epidemiology; the incidence of functionalism and naive sociology in the interpretation of the state and health practices; and the critique of behavioral epistemology that permeated health education and epistemological studies.

It was within that historic epistemological framework that the principal founding works of a different epidemiology appeared. It required an audacious approach to break the conventional dependence on the rigid mold of what Naomar de Almeida-Filho (2000) sharply described as a "timid science" that had passively adopted the empiricist linear canons of causal thinking. We began working on the social determination of health, embedding its explanation in the analysis of production, work, and the conditions of the urban and rural working classes. This was the case for Cristina Laurell's "Sociological Analysis of Morbidity of Two Mexican Peoples"(1976); Cecilia Donnangelo's *Health and Society* (1976); Ana Tambellini's *Work and Disease* (1978); José Carlos Escudero's "Malnutrition in Latin America" (1976); Eduardo Menéndez and his critical anthropological analysis of the surreptitious social cultural determination of the health conceptions and beliefs of communities (1981);and my own work that presented for the first time a clear systematization of the theoretical and methodological proposal for the category of the "social determination of health"— work based on a systematic critique of causal positivism and empirical environmentalism from the perspective of critical realism and political economy (Breilh, 1977).

Those were the first steps in overcoming causal empiricism and the absence of categories with which to analyze the structural basis of the social determination of health and the social contrasts of phenomena in a profoundly unequal society. Parallel efforts were also advancing in the struggle to defeat idealism and functionalist arguments on the state and health policies and behavioral notions on education; overriding contributions were made by such thinkers as Juan Cesar García (1979), an intellectual leader of the movement. It was also the beginning of a critique of the ahistorical conceptions of preventive practice, in which Sergio Arouca—another outstanding inspiratory of our movement— played a fundamental role (Arouca, 1975).

Two postgraduate programs emerged very early in the process: the master's studies program in social medicine at the Autonomous Metropolitan University of Xochimilco in Mexico (1975) and the State University of Rio de Janeiro in Brazil (1976). In addition, the formation of pioneering critical research centers, such as the Center for Health Research and Advisory in Ecuador, was the historical result of this process of debate and conceptual progress. One outstanding step forward in the institutionalization of social medicine was the creation in September 1979 of the Brazilian Association of Postgraduates in Collective Health. Its founders had the resources and political power to put into practice the richness of their national debate and the new Latin American ideas about health. One of its conceptual actions was the formal proposition of collective health as a category for our academic and social identity. This was possible after subjecting to critical scrutiny other terms such as "public health" and "social medicine," thus clarifying the object of transformation that we had fashioned.

In the 1980s, the movement began its second period of diversification: new ways of defining our study objects and subjects, of transforming our academic syllabus, and of reframing our methodology and redesigning our instruments. The intention of all these efforts was the consolidation of the institutional presence of new paradigms. It seems paradoxical to have put such progressive academic transformations into motion precisely when our societies were passing through a decade of aggressive restructuring and adjustment of the productive system, severe legal deregulation, and the demolition of rights and cultural neoconservatism. The strategic avant-garde of the neoliberal project was composed of company representatives and obsequious public servants who pressed to dissolve the role of the state and decentralize its governance. A permanent campaign was implemented with the aim of dismantling social awareness of the collective right to public goods and services. Entrepreneurial lobbying aimed to discredit public solutions as inefficient and expensive and to position the private economy and the market as the perfect sources of health development and social distribution. The result for the working and middle classes was the privatization of public services and social security. Of course, in order to protect the model's hegemony, there was a need to offer low-quality private insurance programs. The so-called universal security system was publicized, with extreme cynicism, as the solution to all the health needs of the poor.

The third and fourth periods of our movement are associated with the challenges of transdisciplinarity (third period in the 1990s) and intercultural meta-critique (fourth period in the new millennium). The paradigm clash of the two previous periods generated new challenges. We not only had to rethink the objects of social medicine but also had to pay more attention to the social subjects of health—both as stakeholders for action and as the subjects of research. This was an opportunity to diversify the study of the social subjects of knowledge. That is, whereas in the formative period of the 1970s, the emphasis was placed on the emancipatory construction of health as an object, circumstances now moved us toward a reworking of health as a subject of praxis. New horizons came into view, and valuable books and articles on gender and ethnicity in health appeared, proposing new methodological instruments to incorporate these into the branches of epidemiology, state theory, knowledge, and communication.

With the turn of the century, the time came to analyze the limiting theoretical and methodological implications of monocultural science. Later, we comment on the historical factors that exerted pressure to incorporate an intercultural scientific viewpoint.

One central challenge of this fourth period has been to examine health problems from a meta-critical perspective. In addition, this endeavor is suitably congruent with the incorporation of the new *objects–subjects* (gender and ethnocultural rights) that had become vital elements of the vision and agenda of collective health and the health rights struggle.

However, one instrumental component of the problem became evident when research groups began to incorporate the qualitative evidence of social change and cultural diversity. Innovate methodology was needed to integrate both quantitative and qualitative components at different stages of knowledge construction.

Unfortunately, in some epistemic scenarios, the critique of quantitative survey empiricism has lent itself to a resurgence of cultural relativism and its new face of qualitative empiricism. However, from a dialectical perspective, the idea has not been to substitute quantitative with qualitative empiricism. The idea was not to operate with those "quali" and "quanti" expressions as fragmented, tip-of-the-iceberg phenomena but, rather, as expressions of concrete embodiments,[5] both qualitative and quantitative, that are generated by a concrete critical process and social determining movement (Breilh, 1997, 2003a). We return to this issue in Chapter 3.

Scholars from different Latin American countries, universities, and social institutions have come together over many decades in order to build the social medicine movement and, more recently, collective health. It has been a counteractive intellectual and political tradition based on a renewed interpretation of health and a participative conception of scientific work. Social medicine has successfully become a driving force in the advance of new ideas and action programs in communities and institutions. This work has entailed important contributions, despite being limited by its subalternate position with respect to mainstream, dominant, and much more generously financed approaches to health science.

---

5. Here, the notion of *embodiment* is used in the sense of giving a concrete perceptible form or body to a process, as explained in Chapter 2, thus expanding Nancy Krieger's (2005, 2011) important definition of *biological incorporation* to the collective (i.e., socionatural) domain.

In the Global North, the historical and vital counterhegemonic traditions of critical public health and social medicine—comparatively stronger in their technical and institutional resources—were, nonetheless, also subordinated to the dominant positivist and functionalist public health paradigm. The driving force of mainstream research with its commoditized science is the economic and political incidence of big biomedical corporations with their unbounded governance over health care, research, and teaching organizations. In general, the biased, lineal, empiricist, and biodeterminist conceptions of health research have directed mainstream resources to the basic sciences and applied clinical and surgical domains. The commercialized health care logic set the pace for all main health-related operations of the field.

Under those conditions, the critical epidemiology paradigm was forced to develop as a counteractive movement, confronting the constraints that hamper its powerful contribution. The alternative paradigm is the result of an articulated set of theoretical, epistemological, methodological, and ethical breaks with hegemonic mainstream epidemiology. I refer to the conceptual core of this innovative science as the *social determination of health*.

Both to the South and to the North of the Rio Grande, peoples are denouncing our ailing world and proposing a profound transformation of our societies. As a result, thousands of public health/collective health researchers and activists who have given the best of their lives to unravel the reality of health in the capitalist world are creatively generating ideas and developing mechanisms for the real protection and promotion of life and human wellness. This is a global movement that stands for the subversion of our unhealthy civilization and for the utopia of good living (enlightened rebelliousness for the 21st century).

2 | WHY CRITICAL EPIDEMIOLOGY?

DARING ETHICAL SCIENCE IN
AN UNHEALTHY CIVILIZATION

Planetary Life Hanging by a Thread: Acceleration of an Unjust and Injurious System

The exponential growth of a discriminatory, rapacious, and oligopolistic market economy in the 21st century is nurtured and reproduced by an unhealthy civilization and its predominant modes of living.

Neoliberal economics, with its absolute belief in the uniquely efficient role of competition in productive optimization and of the market as the optimal distributor and unassailable mechanism of progress, was imposed beginning in the late 1980s. Disregarding a fair distribution of wealth, and dismantling social controls over corporations and the regulatory role of the state over large companies, this aggressive greediness implied the terminal divorce of capitalism from democracy.

At that time, Fukuyama (1989) convinced many people, in the name of neoliberalism, that through capitalism modern civilization had reached the highest peak of development and brought about the end of socio-economic history. However, in the face of the recent global social upheaval and wave of protests, and studies that consistently dismiss Fukuyama's radically biased appraisal, it has been demonstrated that the real symbol of the 21st century is no longer the acceptance of the eternal presence of this highly rapacious economic system but, rather, a growing rejection of extreme inequity and the threat of disappearance (Garcés, 2019).

It is necessary to recognize that some important contradictory nuances have surfaced that add new complexities to the problem. Events such as the recent political upheaval in Brazil and Bolivia and the Ecuadorian and Chilean protests offer new ingredients for our analysis. The growth of social awareness is not monolithic and uniform. The "successful" reforms of progressive governments and even the proclaimed "successes" of right wing neoliberal administrations both point not only to objective institutional and social supposed transformations but also to subjective, cultural, and everyday commonsense structures (Arístegui, 2019). Coming from utterly different social formations, these represent opposing trends that yield vital clues for a deeper understanding of the people's ideology in our contemporary inequitable world.

Denouncing inequality by force of facts has ceased to be a matter for progressive leaders and conscientious investigators and has become the public assertion of conscious grassroots citizens. Beyond the efforts that the powerful have made to hide this growing injustice, the truth is that the people have finally seen what was in plain sight but was not seen due to the game of seductions and backstage bonanzas that had been used to sell them the promise of endless consumerism. And by looking with their own eyes at the reliable materiality of an exponential growth of inequality, whose lethal rhythm is only matched by the astonishing speed of an obscene accumulation of wealth, they are realizing that private capital is "devouring our future" (Piketty, 2015). That significantly reduces collective health improvement opportunities to zero.

The uncontained escalation of multinational corporations is only paralleled by the expanding reduction of spaces for wellness and life. The demolition of social, health, and environmental rights has become a blind pursuit and the principal strategy of big business expansion. This trend is not only present and severely affecting vast numbers of vulnerable communities in the Global South but also impacts many subaltern collectivities of the affluent North.

Present capital accumulation benefits only a minuscule entrepreneurial group. It revolves around the convergence of productivist uses of the technology of the fourth industrial revolution (Ribeiro, 2016); the unfair and fraudulent dispossession of strategic resources in their most varied forms (Harvey, 2003); and even the opportunistic exploitation of conditions of extreme despair, shock, and social anxiety (Klein, 2007). New and aggressive dimensions of technology, hypermedia, and cyberspace also make possible the frenetic expansion of the postmodern consumerist civilization.

The system's striking traditional disparities have widened: The rich to poor income ratio, a universal indicator of inequity, has reached a spine-chilling 1:99% (Open Markets Institute, 2018); research attests to the desperate global migration of the most vulnerable poor, in contrast to the territorial stability of the rich [United Nations (UN), 2017a]; and reports show that small economies are paying a high price, and there is a worldwide violation of the rights of nature due to mega-mining (EJAtlas, 2017) and agribusiness (Cotula, Anseeuw, & Baldinelli, 2019). An unprecedented number of scientific alarm signals related to climate warming populate books and articles, while powerful leaders give resonance to the cynical discourse of climate deniers. In addition, universal violation and commodification of our private lives are made invisible by the expansion of noncritical customers of the networks (Alvaredo, Chancel, Piketty, Saez, & Zucman, 2018; Fry & Taylor, 2018).

The persistent argument of big business is to equate the extreme profit search with progress and the common good. But the saying, "The road to hell is paved with good intentions" has now acquired colossal importance. The prognosticated global trends of economic inequality cast even bigger shadows over the future distribution of wealth. In the view of well-informed analysts, the expanding gap [recapitalization (r) > growth (g): private capital rent > income, production] that existed throughout the 20th century is becoming even greater in the 21st century. According to long trend data, this will be most destabilizing, as the relationship $r > g$ implies that in each new cycle, recapitalization of the past assets is faster than the rate of growth of production and wages.

We witness the historic progress of planetary technology and yet, at the same time, the decomposition of real conditions for social reproduction has reached its greatest level (Arizmendi, 2007). This unabashed recognition of the resounding failure of a civilization in a time of amazing technological potentialities is not only the foremost paradox of the 21st century but also, with regard to health, the principal menace we must face to protect and promote health and natural life.

But to support this finding, it must be understood that the material mechanisms of this unbounded destructiveness and extremely inequitable and unhealthy world system are far from self-sustaining. They are clearly supported in a set of political, cultural, and communicative mechanisms to discipline collectivities and alienate them from their strategic needs. Two types of mechanisms uphold such alienation: renewed cultural hegemony and digitally based cyber subsumption of collective behavior.

The previously submerged and now evident "philosophical war," intended to weaken intercultural relations and install racial/cultural supremacy, is on the run, as has been brilliantly explained by Enrique Dussel, one of Latin America's most lucid contemporary thinkers (Arístegui, 2019). Taking as an example Bolivia's and Brazil's recent political ideological swings, he outlined how a conservative and fundamentalist version of ultra-conservative religious ideology has operated during the past few decades as an instrument of fundamentalist indoctrination. Its aim has been to adapt poor people, through their common sense and profound subjectivity, to the role of functional consumers and defenders of the neoliberal mode of living. The concept of a "new Christ," an "inverse Christianity," not of the poor but of the wealthy, has proliferated through patient grassroots brainwashing. It is a reverse Christianity that disregards or demonizes the ideas of native indigenous peoples and poor communities, seeking to impose the individualist ethos of private wealth building and pragmatic personal success, as modern, superior forms that surpass a supposedly backward communitarianism. This philosophical reversal begins as a means to discredit the sociopolitical ideas of solidarity, equity, and fairness found in Andean or Mezzo American indigenous communities, and it goes on to dismantle a set of ideas and values that make up the powerful heuristic and taxonomies that underlie their sophisticated ecosophical system that protects Nature and places collective rights over individual business.

As explained later, cyber subsumption of collective behavior is impelled and expanded by means of global digital platforms.

Our reflections on social, health, and environmental rights, our contemporary epidemiological notions, can therefore only acquire consistency if we construct them on the body of knowledge and historical experience that criticizes this accelerated entrepreneurial profit building sustained by extremist socially visible or invisible cultural–communicative mechanisms. In order to be imposed, justified, and tolerated, this insatiable accumulation of private wealth with its profit scheme needs to function by means of a combination of force, mass seduction, and a false truth replication apparatus and the violation of all ethical codes, social pacts, and environment agreements. These processes are producing unforeseen massive blows to wellness, collective health conditions, and the environment.

Capital Acceleration 4.0 and Neo-extractivism: Apocalypses or Alert for Transformative Action

To advance its economic apparatus and apply its anthropocentric philosophy, corporations have positioned *extractivism*[1] as the material support of economic expansion (Acosta, 2013). This represents an essential component of an economic system that has endangered the present and future life on Earth due to its extravagant energetic matrix, its wasteful logic, its destructive applications of technology, and its multiplication of inequitable relations.

In the past, extractivism was mainly concentrated on aggressive mechanisms for global control of exportable nonrenewable goods production (i.e., metal mining and oil and agricultural products). Capital accumulation demands highly specialized and continuous large-scale production processes. And in the case of the enormous territories of agricultural extractivism, it involves control over vast territories, water and seeds, and, more recently, genetic resources and artificial biology. For many years, land grabbing was the principal mechanism for installing profitable low-cost production processes through immense, monotonous one-crop landscapes. It became the key path to territorial control. The history of neocolonialism shows that it is based on

---

1. "Extractivism is the process of extracting natural resources from the Earth to sell on the world market. It exists in an economy that depends primarily on the extraction or removal of natural resources that are considered valuable for exportation worldwide. Some examples of resources that are obtained through extraction include gold, diamonds, lumber and oil" (Acosta, 2013).

land grabbing. In the case of Liberia, for example, the arrival of the Firestone Rubber Company at the beginning of the 20th century initiated the violent transition from a family-based agrarian economy to an entrepreneurial export economy. The company took possession of approximately half a million hectares for 99 years, at 6 cents for every 0.40 hectares. The story of how 20,000 indigenous people living in this area were forced to work on the Firestone plantations is painful evidence of the negative effects of agro-industrial greed (Hancock, 2017). Large companies have been striving to take possession of immense and ever-growing territories, either by global land purchase transactions (Nolte, Chamberlain, & Giger, 2016) or by leasing (Hahn, 2012). Throughout the world, this type of extreme rapacity has changed little in recent times.

In geographical terms, land use maps of the region show the decrease of biosphere reserves, the expansion of oil exploration blocks and mega-mining concessions in protected areas, as well as the impacts on agricultural areas resulting from the implantation of agro-industrial and mining enclaves.

From that insensitive, shortsighted, and opportunistic perspective, biodiverse multiple crop territories are viewed as economically inefficient. According to that paradoxical reasoning, "what is important for a sustainable planet is an obstacle to efficient extraction" and "biodiversity amounts to bad corporate business" (Bartra, 2006). The problem is that exponential growth of that type of agribusiness is an attack on all human rights. The problem is out of control, to the point that the UN Special Rapporteur on the right to food straightforwardly declared in relation to pesticide application (UN, 2017b)—one of the lethal elements—that

> pesticides impose substantial costs on Governments and have catastrophic impacts on the environment, human health and society as a whole, implicating a number of human rights and putting certain groups at elevated risk of rights abuses. . . . Harm to the ecosystem presents a considerable challenge. This challenge has been exacerbated by a systematic denial, fuelled by the pesticide manufacturers and agro-industries. (p. 4)

The logic of mega-extraction is oriented toward whatever operations prove most profitable. In recent times, the decline of oil prices and the global recognition of environmental contamination caused by fossil fuels have placed great pressure on the current oil-based production and energy system. The current global mining extractivist boom likely owes its impetus to this crisis. Open-pit mining concessions are soaring, and countries are paying a high price for the global mineral boom, especially those of the Global South (Siegel, 2013). To accompany its global boom, mega-mining has also incorporated risky high-tech procedures (Vidal & Guest, 2015). The entrepreneurial argument is that "the internet of things, robotics and plasma are transforming mining into a safer and more productive industry" (Mining Technology, 2014).

However, in the past few years, extraction has expanded to encompass new productive technologies that accelerate capital accumulation, reduce production costs, and allow the production of an entirely new set of high-demand commodities. To do so, capitalism's fourth industrial revolution has led to an explosive convergence of new technologies. An array of applications in robotics, nanotechnology, biotechnology, big data operations, hypermedia, and artificial intelligence constitute a powerful industrial arsenal (Ribeiro, 2016).

In addition to the better known applications of nanotechnology, genetic engineering, and informatics in fields such as medicine and agriculture, the newer and less studied operation of digital global platforms, which extract people's data and turn mega personal databases into extremely lucrative merchandise, is a new flourishing type of extractivism (Subirats, 2019). Such is the importance of cyber production that in the world's largest economy, two firms own 97% of the market share of search engines: Alphabet (91%) and Microsoft (6%) (Open Markets Institute, 2018). As in the rest of the world, in Latin America huge corporate digital platforms extract the personal data of millions of computer and smartphone users (e.g., Facebook, Instagram, and Twitter), or data are obtained through the instantaneous connection of millions of consumers by service providers that operate through apps (e.g., Uber Eats, Seamless, and Door Dash). For instance, shared mobility in Latin America is the second fastest growing mobile market: In 2018, revenue generated by ride-hailing apps in the region was $518 million, and it is expected to increase to more than $1 billion by 2023. Uber entered the Latin American carshare market in 2013 and, according to its records, currently has more than 36 million active users (Phillips, 2018).

If we put aside for a moment the circumstantial individual practical benefits of those platforms and enquire about the massive negative socio-epidemiological implications of their current wide-scale operations, we come to understand the contradictory role of cybernetic processes in the social determination of our modes of living, the workplace, and our rights and health. In my keynote speech to the 9th Brazilian Congress of Epidemiology (held at the Federal University of Espírito Santo in 2014) published in the *Brazilian Journal of Epidemiology* (Breilh, 2015b), I stated,

> The new digital technological revolution, about which some frightening prognoses are made for the next decades, could easily imply the advent of an era of radical subsumption of life processes. This will negatively affect not only our general way of living, thinking and planning, but also our deepest daily intimacy. This movement implies radical effects on health that we call cybernetic determination and subsumption. This novel process raises new questions on public health and prevention; but also requires a new reading of reality, a rethinking of human life and health, of its social determination, which implies the need for new categories and analysis and renewed challenges for critical epidemiology. (p. 945)

A range of health-related processes have emerged within the cyber domain in this new epoch. An illustrative problem is the unprecedented impact of cyber production on work, labor, and health rights. In the case of ride-hailing services such as Uber, Cabify, and others, the transnational firms control the performance and locations of their supposedly "self-employed" drivers through maximum monitoring algorithms. On the basis of their power to substitute drivers immediately and unilaterally, in most countries these virtual workers operate at their own risk, without contract or labor rights. Labor inequity is the rule given that the companies assign workers different salaries according to seasonal conditions. Asymmetries of power, biased access to information, and "hidden" unsafe working conditions are the governing rule. The companies' gigantic digital platform algorithms allow them to connect providers and demanding citizens as an intermediary; the companies do not need to own the products that are sold, the instruments, or the vehicles. Nor are the employees under contract with the companies; they are "autonomous entrepreneurs," but in reality they are not "self-employed" workers because they are tightly regulated in the intensely monitored and generally risky labor operations the companies control.

In the past few decades, a dark episode of health-related scientific fraud—that has immense public health consequences—occurred in the field of genetic engineering; this episode helps us understand the consequences of corporate pressure on science—pressure that endangers human and natural health. The plainly depicted and widely documented case of false evaluation and the consequent dismissal of the real risks of the genetic insertion of recombinant DNA (rDNA) in the *Escherichia coli* K12 bacteria triggered an alarm in the academic world about the dangerous effects of so-called *molecular politics*. Three closed-door national meetings held to evaluate the safety of genetically modified organisms (GMOs)(Bethesda, MD, in 1976; Falmouth, MA, in 1977; Ascot, UK, in 1978) and the Cohen report on the safety of rDNA (S. Wright, 1994) concealed important concerns and uncertainties about genetic modification that were circulating in the academic community, and it mistakenly concluded that there was enough consistent research on GMO safety (Druker, 2013).

In this emblematic case, a triple fraud has been suggested: (1) giving the impression that the insertion of a foreign gene into another organism was a natural process;(2) the generation of a belief that proteins codified by a foreign gene are adequately expressed; and(3) that this sort of experiment works well with all vegetable and animal genes, when in fact it only worked with non-inhibitory mitochondrial genes[2] (Druker, 2013). In the case of rDNA, not only were certain scientific procedures inadvertently altered behind closed doors, with the support of a public agency, but also essential genetic regulation mechanisms were intentionally altered.

The fact that in plants the genetic obstacles are even more complex, and gene insertion faces stronger physiologic defenses, encouraged different ways to penetrate plants' organic barriers and promote their genetic expression. The following are milestones in the development of genetically modified food: bacterial insertion of *Agrobacterium tumefaciencis* that was able to misinform the plant in order to express its own genes (Latham, Wilson, & Steinbrecher, 2006; Reese, 2006, pp. 46–47); the development of promoters of genetic expression (e.g., 35s promoter), and particle bombardment or bio-ballistics that penetrates corn cells

---

2. Because bacteria cannot adequately express the genes of higher animals due to the fact that it is not able to deal with introns, different types of enzymatic promoters, terminators, and codons, the genetic engineers removed the introns; they avoided codons and replaced them with others manageable by bacteria. Also, they did not include promoter and terminator sequences but instead put their synthetic gene under the control of a bacterial promoter and terminator. All this happened without sufficient knowledge or proof of unpredictable consequences (Druker, 2013).

with foreign DNA (Kneen, 1999, p. 26). The search for valuable corn and soy crops in which to employ genetic enhancement was intense.

During this quest for improved productivity, unpredictable and uncontrolled results were amply documented in specialized literature. It demonstrates a flagrant sophism with regard to the boundless benefits of business-applied high tech. Along the way, scientific and legal rejection of the argument that genetic engineering innocuously replicates natural processes has proved that the "venture to genetically engineer our food has subverted science, corrupted governance and systematically deceived the public" (Druker, 2013, p. 60).

The panacea of technological manipulation of nature is applied for purposes of profit without sufficient experimental testing, in a manner that impedes both the application of the precautionary principle (Breilh, 2018a) and the democratic surveillance of its potential or actual risks. The same applies to climate engineering by means of the injection of aerosols in the stratosphere; the brightening of oceanic clouds to increase rainfall in agricultural territories (Straffon, 2018); or neuronal networks, machine learning, deep learning, as well as artificial biology, which are being developed by corporate researchers and "philosophers." Contracted groups build algorithms for entrepreneurial applications of artificial intelligence in a diversity of disciplinary fields, such as economics and biology (Rodriguez-Beltrán, 2018). Automated decision-making systems embody socially determined political, ethnic, gender, and other preconceptions, which are contained on the huge data sets that serve for their "training." This *algorithm bias* encompasses immense threats with respect to technological objectivity and neutrality (Naughton, 2019) and is becoming the accelerator of 21st-century racism and social exclusion. System 2 reasoning permits going beyond cognition linked to very concrete situations to understanding underlying structures at a very deep level. Giant database handling, at speeds that surpass human capabilities, has allowed for the placement of artificial simulation of natural neuronal and biological fluxes in artificial people and animals that can greatly exceed the cognitive and physical powers that nature has provided: "artificial creatures that—in suitable contexts—appear to be persons or animals" (Bringsjord & Govindarajulu, 2018).

The development of artificial life beyond the current natural reality, with its clear potential to change and challenge what we have recognized as human and natural life up to now, has resulted in some epistemologists, philosophers, ethicists, and anthropologists coining terms such as "posthumanism." This represents a recent movement that can be viewed from different perspectives: criticizing classical humanism, condemning the anthropocentric perspective that commoditizes natural processes, or proposing to go beyond the protection of humans and recognize the need to defend all living beings against exponentially accelerated transformative processes. An extreme, desperate, outlook proposes the need to confront a so-called human demise in a terminal era of a supposed "end of humanity," in which artificial creatures take over operations and decision-making in crucial areas of our cities, mines, and agro-industries (Ferrando, 2013). New technologies in the control of big business are inevitably leading humanity to a regressive revolution. Their marvelous potentialities are kidnapped and submitted to the logic of domination and profit.

The groundbreaking potential of artificial intelligence is also leading the system to what has been called the philosophical revolution of artificial life and intelligence. The dubious discourse of technologically based *singularity* forms part of the intellectual climate that is created around artificial intelligence. Singularity relates to the new immortal state that would be reached when artificial intelligence surpasses human intelligence. Mainly signifying the new capitalist nirvana of artificially designed people, technological convergence would make this possible, where nano- and biotechnologies are the hardware of the new artificial life, and informatics and cognitive technologies are its software (Cordeiro, 2019). Even discarding the veracity of these suppositions, the debate about a final "singularity" designed by the philosophers of big companies now forms part of the 21st-century episteme. Human standards for similarity based on a controlled pattern of traits would form part of an entrepreneurial utopia. It would aim to demolish the utopian democratic construction of a world of diversity. The current and future dispute over the control of technology will determine the fate of humanity and wellness.

We must also be aware of what artificial life and intelligence, in the wrong hands, can do in the present not only to physical health and environmental conditions but also to the philosophical and material foundations of society. The distribution of high-tech research resources is intensely inequitable and is destined to expand already pronounced social and cultural gaps.

Finally, it is important not to lose sight of an apparent contradiction that has become a 21st-century paradox: an unleashed market monopoly combined with pre-capitalist agricultural relations to complete the extraction scheme. Big business' control of land, technology, and cheap labor has become even more profitable and competitive through unfair social and market relations and powerful lobbying. High-tech-based inequity combines with historic pre-capitalist overtly rapacious labor exploitation. Millions of "independent" small producers are submitted to disadvantageous production and market relations and policies or are invited to join the scheme as associated low-cost providers of certain subcomponents. Under these opportunistic mechanisms, the lower production costs of large high-tech estates entail prejudicial competition with small family farmers and present the additional benefit of differential rent for agribusiness (Bartra, 2008).

The resultant corollary of this vitiated structure that favors an unsustainable, plundering, and harmful agricultural system on the planet is that more than 1.5 billion peasant families and indigenous farmers, who together with 410 million gatherers in forests, jungles, and savannahs generate between 70% and 80% of the world's food (Rosset & Altieri, 2019), are forced to operate in extremely disadvantageous conditions. Rapacious businessmen, their political partners, and scientific henchmen such as climate deniers seem to underestimate that sooner or later all this irrationality will strike back and the historical pendulum will swing, as is demonstrated by the massive youth mobilizations in Europe and the people's anti-neoliberal protests in Chile and Ecuador.

The resounding voice of the International Peasants Movement (Via Campesina), a global movement that comprises more than 182 organizations in 81 countries with 200 million affiliates, is speaking for all of us when it denounces this "acceleration to disaster." The only viable and effective way to build a global movement for a clean and just food system and to put in place consistent health prevention and promotion strategies is to build a hands-on international platform to fully support the organizations and small family and cooperative medium-scale units that apply agro ecological, healthy, and sustainable farming (International Peasants Movement, 2008).

Cities also make up part of this troubled planet. The ecosystem and epidemiological setbacks are also urban. Here, we not only refer to deteriorating indexes of pollutants such as airborne particles that contribute to causing cancers and lung and heart disease, and also cause adverse effects on fetal development and foster poor lung and brain development in children. These are deteriorating, of course, not only in peripheral Third World cities but also in cities such as London, where ultra-fine particles resulting from vehicle emissions, domestic heating, and industrial pollution have reached extremely high levels—more than double the World Health Organization (WHO) standard of 10 µg.[3] We must pay closer attention to what has been called "savage urbanism," which constitutes the quintessence of urban capital acceleration in the *neoliberal city*. The poisonous cocktail of this process is the wholesale privatization of services, the construction of a real estate bubble for income extraction, the uncontrolled absorption of the poor expelled from the countryside by growing slums, and the expansion of dangerous neighborhoods (Barreda, 2008). Opportunistic

---

3. According to Professor Annette Peters, Director of the Institute of Epidemiology at the Helmholtz Zentrum, Munich, interviewed by *The Guardian* on December 14, 2019 (https://www.theguardian.com/environment/2019/dec/14/uk-must-limit-killer-ultra-fine-air-pollutants?CMP=share_btn_link).

gentrification and segregation of urban facilities and services according to postal code is constantly denounced by peoples' organizations as a potent sign of regressive urban legislation.

Municipal spatiality, distribution, mobility, and landscapes are determined by an accelerated, unconsult, disorderly, and unhealthy logic that has generated the urban face of the global crisis. Cities' development is implemented in order to benefit business enclaves and to segregate the extremely luxurious and overserviced habitats of the rich; the well-provided settings of the middle class; the deficient, contaminated, and perilous municipal locations of worker neighborhoods; and the ever-growing chaotic, extremely insecure, and overcrowded slums of the subproletarian population. Latin American epidemiology has documented the significant epidemiological differentials that have appeared in neoliberal cities (Barata, Barreto, Almeida-Filho, & Veras, 1997; Behm, 1992; Breilh, Granda, Campaña, & Betancourt, 1983; Bronfman, 1992; C. García, 1986).

Mega processes have resulted in planetary life and health hanging by a thread, by damaging and distorting the construction of sustainable, sovereign, solidary, and safe societies; to make things worse, they have concomitantly favored and sometimes even triggered the aberrant expressions of terrorism and the narcotics business. For instance, the poisonous penetration of narcotics business ventures is devouring the institutional ethos of our societies. Operating by means of different platforms and corridors, they have achieved varying degrees of infiltration of the sociopolitical scenarios of the South and North, no matter the political model. Having the affluent North as the big buyer, narcotics businesses have operated at times from Colombia, at times from

Russia, and now principally from Mexico, using different countries either as transportation corridors or as marketplaces. This has signified the establishment of narcotics production and trafficking territories and corridors, often in association with the morally decayed dissidents of guerrilla organizations that historically arose as liberation armies.

This historical shift of 21st-century civilization under the powerful umbrella of huge multinational corporations represents a global blow to the possibilities for collective and public health. It has shaken the philosophical and ethical foundations of the market society. This colossal setback of humanity challenges all of us working in the life sciences.

The Downfall of Common Good and Derailment of Institutional Ethos

The demanding, honorable, and benevolent practices of epidemiology in sanitary posts and in a diversity of public and private health, teaching, and research units throughout the world comprise a formidable and dignified dossier. However, as members of today's globalized societies, epidemiologists are, willingly or unwillingly, hostages to the civilization we have just profiled. They must carry on limited preventive and health promotion activities in communities and workplaces that form part of cities and regions that endure a new alienated logic of living, in which the historical essentials of formerly progressive unionism have been derailed, servile or limited functional forms of organization prevail for the moment, and the positive action of valuable activist fronts and organizations is systematically offset by the fear and conservatism of silent majorities. The alienating winners–losers philosophy that rewards irresponsible consumerist individualism and punishes concerned communitarianism is the rule of a suicidal game.

So we all strive for health in an era in which public governance cynically tolerates health inequity and absorbs decadent forms of individualism, colonialism, and sexism either at home or abroad. Our societies are forced to maneuver in the frantic rhythms of functional and fearful modes of living that operate in spaces designed to prop up the system and enhance functional living codes, while health professionals must deal with a tsunami of unhealthy, destructive processes that lessen the protective effects of their benevolent and supportive actions. The premonitory argument of Hannah Arendt (1968) that a never-ending accumulation of property must be based on a never-ending accumulation of power is clearly reasserted by the present exacerbation of the apparatus of political dominance.

It is now clearer than ever that the ethical–cultural dimension, the frenetic expansion of postmodern consumerist civilization, is reproducing and confirming the prophesy made by Pasolini in his "Corsair Writings," published in 1975, in which he denounces the coming of a new fascism that replaces violent methods with the self-imposed domination of consumerist ideology—a process that "is not humanistically rhetorical, but Americanly pragmatic. Its purpose is the reorganization and brutally totalitarian homologation of the world" (International Peasants Movement, 2008, p. 6).

And as part of this global regression, a rapacious neocolonialism is expanding and intensifying.

For those of us who work for the protection and promotion of life, the major contradiction of the 21st century is that we live in a context of historically unprecedented technological potential and renewed cultural diversity—traits that constitute powerful and promising possibilities for the common good—while at the same time being subject to the material basis of a deadly economy and the philosophical basis of a global ethical setback.

Climate change is the tip of the iceberg of the environmental hecatomb that is submerging capitalist postmodern societies of the fourth industrial revolution in behaviors that are "incompatible with the configuration of the world of life itself" (Echeverría, 2015, p. 51). We are immersed in a new cannon of the organization of life, both practical and intellectual, which has three main characteristics: an unrestricted devotion to technical capability based on the cold use of reason, the secularization of the political sphere (political materialism) expressed as the preeminence of shortsighted economic policy, and the aforementioned centrality of individual desires (Echeverría, 2015).

If we analyze Echeverría's (2015) philosophical assertion from an epidemiological perspective, we can expect very serious consequences for the fabrication of utopia and for the construction of healthy, sustainable, and caring societies. Taken together, the unbridled advance of a technologically accelerated material base of exploitation, the expansion of a radically individualistic, technocratic, and secularized civilization, the increasing dedication of social space for the benefit of major private interests, and the intensification of colonialism imply the defeat of the common good and the imposition of a new geography of inequity, exclusion, and death. This represents three negative trends.

First is a downfall of the sacred vision of the world and its natural spaces that has submerged nations in the profane and pragmatic trend of extractivist projects. We are experiencing and accepting the substitution of the accumulated social wisdom of First Nations and peasants with respect to Mother Nature by a shortsighted pragmatic reason that mathematizes nature and territories in order to use them for the extraction of private profit.

The expanded anthropogenic destruction of nature and human health is generally disguised by production mechanisms that are presented as correct, safe, and ecologically sensitive but that in practice take on a brutal form. The barbarian bonfire that agribusiness, landowners, and ignorant political leaders have ignited and promoted of late in the Amazon not only denotes extreme cynicism and scientific illiteracy but also constitutes painful, mind-boggling proof of the veracity of our argument that terrestrial life is hanging by a thin and fragile thread. In this case, the vital planetary metabolism of water, climate regulation, and oxygen production that is supported by 600 billion Amazon trees, the ecosophical communities and women who protect life, the animals, vegetation, and microscopic life that sustain natural cycles is currently being destroyed at an alarming rate by a handful of greedy companies and ill-informed landowners in the name of progress.

In Lefebvrian terms (Lefebvre, 2007), we must admit that national and international territories are no longer a sphere for an all-encompassing social and natural reproduction but, rather, have become spaces of aggressive capital accumulation (Harvey, 2007) at the expense of all forms of life and ethical principles. The concrete geographical expression of this process is that rural and urban spaces are no longer places essentially dedicated to produce *use values* (food and other goods), under effective regulations and basic codes for social protection and rights. What we now have is an urban–rural fracture, in which unleashed productivist greed operates to produce commodities with a competitive *exchange value* in order to generate profit rather than producing goods with strategic use value for the reproduction of humans and all living beings (Echeverria, 2017).

Second is a decline in political spiritualism that degrades the value of politics as a tool for developing rights, solidarity links for effective social agency, and cultural means for the reproduction of identity. This moral and practical shift of politics at the hands of the powerful imposes the supremacy of private profit and interests. The political mission, for and from the territories, now ignores the ethical and the fight for territory as a space of emancipation and identity, rather assuming these as arenas of hegemony and the political technocratic control of private interests.

Third is a profound setback for the decolonized communitarian philosophy that originally characterized the human being, together with its remnants of collective sociability, with the consequent imposition of private interests on individually owned and colonized spaces. According to this logic, the construction of spaces based on the philosophy of the common good is discarded in order to impose geography of the productive, defensive, and classist enclosure of private ventures, and corresponding areas of extraction, commerce, and mobility.

Nonetheless, the democratic, benevolent side of humanity fortunately keeps producing potent ideas with which to untangle and undo the disarray. Throughout the world, we find expressions of social wisdom and massive global mobilizations that denounce the dreadful wrongdoings of a decadent capitalist system. Gender, ethnic, human rights, youth, and environment–climate activists, artists for health, teachers and scientists, urban and rural workers, and millions of youthful scholars represent the moral reserve of this sick planet. The urgent need to redirect the powerful potential of knowledge, dignity, and wisdom motivates millions of health workers and many epidemiologists to fuel the torch of good living and meta-critical[4] awareness on the planet, waiting for a profound change of our social system and its civilization.

Myths of "Progressive" Technocracy (Aberration of Health Governance): The "Sins of Expertness"

As explained previously, the rapid global shift to a high-tech-based economy that has taken place since the beginning of this century has modernized and accelerated the neoliberal scheme, with serious repercussions for the North–South geopolitical balance.

In recent decades, Latin America, as other regions of the Global South, has lived in hope of democratization and decolonization.

---

4. *Metacritic* is a notion that encompasses intercultural and transdisciplinary counter-hegemonic action that the author has developed as the essential guideline of emancipatory epidemiological action; it is further explained in Chapter 3.

Collective health advocates with different social and ideological perspectives cherished the appearance of new horizons for justice and wellness. In some countries, such as Chile and Colombia, the neoliberal model persisted throughout the past decades with macroeconomic indicators producing a false image of untrammelled progress. Chile is an emblematic example of the inconsistency of neoliberal hegemony and the inevitable contradiction between aggressive private capital accumulation and social wellness. On the other hand, the electoral success of so-called progressive governments in some countries triggered an era of social–democratic hopes. Within the capitalist framework, certain limited social advances were achieved: the implementation of minor redistributive processes; the relative reversion of the dominance of the neoliberal market over the public domain; and the emergence of UNASUR (the alternative Union of South American Nations) as a form of integration opposed to the geopolitical logic of asymmetrical, disadvantageous free trade agreements. In these countries, anti-establishment rhetoric came to the fore of political discourse, ushering in a climate of progressiveness and recovery of sovereignty and justice. Advances were undoubtedly made toward equitable territorial management and the creation of areas of affirmative action that favored communities and some minorities. But with the passage of time, willingly or not, potentially democratic undertakings dissolved into changes that preserved and even consolidated the established order.

The practices of extractivism intercepted the progression of rights advocacy and public services development, restraining them and disrupting the ethical standards of public servants. Oil extraction, mining, and agribusiness were presented as the golden rule for achieving progress and profitable governance in countries with an abundance of valuable natural resources. In order to conceal the inevitable social and environmental consequences, the notion of "good extractivism"[5] had to be disseminated by the propaganda apparatus. The construction of hegemony in those muddy grounds implied a form of governance that reaffirmed and legitimized the model by distancing itself in the public's memory from the openly neoliberal privatization policies of previous years. Switching from market-centered policies to a public investment state model focused on aggressive public infrastructure development and administrative modernization policies initially fostered hegemony. This clearly happened in fields of social interest such as education (school building), health (construction of medical care units), and transportation (road building), in which the public investment curve increased considerably. Second, fresh funds were provided to the populist distribution of social welfare bonuses, using these to build a clientele and political support network.

This demanded a judicial and institutional shift that would accommodate powerful international corporations and national big business within the logic of the state-centered model. Unfortunately, in some cases the persistent thirst for resources derailed the ethics of public administration and well-intentioned redistributive policies. The sky-high prices of key export commodities, and the corresponding plenitude of public funds in the hands

---

5. In a manner that reminds us of the recent debates on fake political truth, the discourse of "good" extractivism that pays for social expenditures, that has become common during the past two decades, especially among these self-proclaimed "progressive" Latin American governments.

of key decision-makers, created a breeding ground for straightforward corruption or, in some cases, the appropriation of public
funds to finance the political apparatus.

History will inevitably confirm or deny the veracity and extent of the claims of corruption that proliferated around these
governments. Nevertheless, it is a fact that bulky dossiers have
been presented and accusations made; history will clarify if they
were bogus political constructs or the genuine derailment of
governments with initially democratic aspirations. Whatever the
case, perverse mechanisms bled or drained the national treasury,
leaving a residual crisis that is now being used to justify an exacerbation of the neoliberal cycle. The process we are describing
consequently led to a "rescue," designed to fix the misdeeds of
an entire decade, with policies such as those promoted by the
International Monetary Fund, whose typical methods leave devastating consequences—as we learned in the case of Greece—with
measures placed on the shoulders of the poorest and provoking
serious consequences for labor rights, services, and epidemiology
(Inman & Smith, 2013).

From an integral social wellness perspective, one can understand that aside from some temporal improvements in income
and living conditions, the driving force of extractivism induced
dubious governance and a systematic distortion of social and
public health development actions. It also endorsed the opportunistic and secular political philosophy we previously analyzed and
assumed communities as clientele to be bought.

What we have now is the underlying contradictions of thriving
neoliberal cities with fashionable neighborhoods and continuously
growing slums, a rural environment with booming agribusiness

and poor working-class communities, regions with an exponential increase in the automotive fleet used for private and business transport, and ever shrinking safe transportation for the poor. These, among other controversial realities of the neoliberal iceberg, confirm an unprecedented reproduction and amplification of social inequity and unhealthy modes of living in segregated, contaminated, insecure dwelling places.

Understanding this complex global regression is crucial to comprehend the multidimensional processes that determine collective epidemiological conditions. The social determination of wellness and health, the subsumption of the biological world in the social world (Breilh, 1977, 2003a), and, correspondingly, the specific forms of what has been defined as corporal and mental embodiments (Krieger, 2005, 2011) can only be understood when their analysis is inserted in a broader contextual determination.

In epidemiological terms, what we find in our countries as a result of this modality of social reproduction is an increase of two principal morbidity profiles: disorders that are more prevalent in subaltern non-entrepreneurial impoverished urban and rural populations (i.e., caloric protein malnutrition; diabetes; old, emergent, and reemerging transmissible diseases, including old and new forms of vector-borne diseases; and certain neoplasms such as of the uterine cervix) and those that are mostly prevalent in modernized industrial and consumerist enclaves (i.e., obesity; chemical precursor and radiation pulmonary neoplasms; leukemia; work overload and stress disorders; immunity disorders; addictions; and anorexia, bulimia, tanorexia, and multiple toxicity disorders) (Breilh, 2010).

Unfortunately, the just demands of affected communities and concerned citizens fall on the deaf ears of the facto illiterate powerful. We can profile this typical pattern with some illustrative examples. In North America, the devastating impacts of oil fracking (hydraulic fracturing) and the severe pollution of the water system in Flint, Michigan (Pauli, 2019), capture the role of big business denial confronted by victimized communities. In Asia, the case of privatization and total drainage and rupture of the natural cycle of aquifer recovery in an important region such as Plachimada (Kerala, India) can only be understood in the framework of unfair and fraudulent concessions to soft drink producers (Bijoy, 2018) that keep recycling their devastating production mechanisms in different locations. In South America is the equally emblematic and alarming expansion of gigantic genetically modified soy plantations in the Southern Cone countries (Melón & Zuberman, 2014), bravely contested in the case of Argentina by the women of the Ituzaingo Movement. The forest fires set in order to establish oil or agro industrial enclaves in Brazil (Escobar, 2019) or the struggle and repression of the Ecuadorian Amazonian communities protesting against oil concessions in one of the world's most biodiverse (supposedly protected) areas of the planet are other examples. All these cases exhibit the same logic of siege and final dispossession in favor of corporations that have operated in collusion with governments, even those of the self-denominated progressive variety.

The golden years of state-centered "progressivism," with its socially amicable narrative, large public investment, middle-class public employment, and aid for the extremely poor, came to an end when the market prices of commodities suffered a critical decline. The crisis revealed that the model had trapped countries in a perverse logic that was paradoxically turning their abundance into impoverishment and growing debt (Breilh & Tillería Muñoz, 2009). This type of techno-bureaucratic management not only left the power of the old ruling classes untouched, or even increased it, but also nurtured forms of accumulation of a new bourgeoisie based on the appropriation of public assets.

Overall and beyond the permanent rhetoric of responsible governance, the practice of extractivism has circumvented constitutional obligations and legal regulations, restraining the role of the state as the constitutional guarantor of human, social, cultural, health, and environmental rights. On the planning tables of diligent members of the powerful bureaucracy, community demands for the reinforcement of safeguards for protected territories and conservational constitutional rights are being overtly described as obstacles to "progress."

The experience of common people has made clear that the mythical discourse of "socially justified extractivism" was merely a set of instrumental statements with which to build political support. The media and many technical reports highlighted the growth of per capita public health investment (i.e., hospitals, health centers, and personnel) and the increases in budget funds that accrued to the sector, assuming at the same time that the modest decline of some basic mortality rates was a sign of successful performance of the populist model. Unfortunately, when one looks at the statistical panorama, it does not show consistent improvement, and in many cases it denotes deteriorating patterns (Breilh, 2018a). Sharpening the contradiction both in the North and in the South, "an increasingly transnational corporate health care industry . . . aggressively aims to exploit the gaps left open by underfunded or nonexistent public provision, furthering commodification and fragmentation" (Waitzkin et al., 2018, p. 239).

People have learned the lesson. Capital investment that benefits the medical industry apparatus does not generate consistent improvement of health indicators. Although the financing and modernizing of conventional public health care installations and the increase in professional resources have partially improved the old health care system, the potentially favorable impact of this policy has been counteracted by the low quality of such investments and the proliferation of unhealthy processes under conditions imposed by the destructive nature of the development model.

At the same time, the prevention and surveillance organisms are weak and ineffective and have become functional to the biomedical hegemonic system. Paradoxically, in years of higher per capita health investment, vaccination coverage in Ecuador declined by 25% between 2009 and 2017, and the country had the worst performance in Latin America (Aguilar, 2019). In fact, crucial protection coverage indicators tumbled, and the 116–120% coverage normally achieved before 2006 declined for all vaccines (Equipo Evaluador Internacional, 2017).

The "sins of expertness" are part of this paradoxical social and health system with its technocratic governance. The vertical foreign certification and evaluation systems that have been imposed on productive, educational, and services provision venues become normative straightjackets for universities, nongovernmental organizations, research units, etc. As a noted researcher declared, programs and projects are subject to arbitrary decisions because "reviewers face the unavoidable temptation to accept or reject new evidence and ideas, not on the basis of their scientific merit, but on the extent to which they agree or disagree with the public positions taken by experts on these matters" (Sackett, 2000, p. 1283). Biased rejection operates in conscious of unconscious manners against new or contesting ideas.

Correspondingly, we must raise our academic-informed voices to challenge the unfairness and destructiveness of our societies and their health establishment demanding a "paradigm shift . . . requiring changes in how we train, reward, promote, and fund the generation of health scientists who will be tasked with breaking out of their disciplinary silos to address this urgent constellation of health threats" (Myers, 2018, p. 2860; see also Dunk, Jones, Capon, & Anderson, 2019).

This global setback presents people, leaders, intellectuals, and scientists with new challenges. It constitutes a moral and organizational tour de force that places extreme pressure on the wisdom, creativity, organizational strength, and technical skills of all the people, both academic and social, as well as the gender, ethnic, and cultural organizations that are permanently mobilized throughout the world, inspired by the utopian principle that another world is possible.

What Makes Transformative Audacious Health and Life Sciences?

So far, we have profiled the historic reasons for the current need for critical, transformative, and ethically audacious health and life sciences. A much-needed global academic mobilization to defend endangered life and accompany the global movement to forward human multicultural knowledge to confront the menaces and develop real solutions.

Virchow's (1848) arguments that preserving health and preventing disease requires full and unlimited democracy and radical measures rather than mere palliatives is more relevant than ever. But one should add that radical (i.e., critical) measures require radical thinking and methodology. In many fields—and epidemiology is no exception—scientific reform is lagging behind the current material and spiritual challenges of an expectant humanity. The health field is profoundly penetrated by the Cartesian logic. Rigor and complex thinking have been reduced to sophistication of quantitative empirical reasoning.

There are two important aspects of critical thinking. Foucault relates it to the capacity to deconstruct and reinvent epistemological certainties; discern and unveil mechanisms of coercion of knowledge; question the politics of truth and question truth as it operates through power; and go beyond the limits that hinder one's subjecthood (Foucault, Lotringer, & Hochroth, 2007). These traits are fundamental to the work of all conscientious scholars. However, as previously explained, in revealing the mechanisms of coercion and interrogating the politics of truth, it is also important to understand the profound epistemological relation between scientific modeling; the dominant paradigms that mold it; and the hidden cultural rules (episteme), pressures, and obstacles exercised by the power structure of society.

When elucidating how "humans are made subjects" and the "modes of objectification that transform human beings into subjects," Foucault (1982) explained the incidence of power relations that dominant states have institutionalized as a convenient form of official science. It is a methodology that ends up supporting a way of ordering the world according to the prevailing conditions of acceptability. This is possible because the explanatory authority of science and the practical power of technology are powerful tools for mastery and social control. Whether for practical productive purposes or for ideological reasons, knowledge is basic to the construction of hegemony. And it is precisely at this point that the functional paradigm of official conventional epidemiology is revealed.

In these circumstances, one most serious epistemological problem that academic communities face is that although a growing number of researchers have voiced their disagreement with the interpretative limitations of positivism and its functional role, and despite the fact that logical *empiricism*[6] has been questioned in important academic circles, it continues to exercise a heavy influence on scientific work in many places, especially in mainstream science (Boltvinik, 2005). In effect, empirical experience based on direct observation being the supposed inductive fundament of all knowledge and having reduced theorizing to inference on related empirical phenomena (Punch, 2016) converts science, as we discuss later, in a mere reflection of empirical tip-of-the-iceberg facts and relations, renouncing to the complex understanding of crucial processes of the real world that have a concrete existence but are not directly perceivable. To say that a research question has to be

---

6. "Empiricism is a philosophical term to describe the epistemological theory that regards experience as the foundation or source of knowledge" (Aspin, 1995).

an empirical question amounts to saying that we would have to answer it only and fundamentally by means of direct, observable tangible facts, qualitative or quantitative, renouncing to empirical phenomena that do not appear as significant—according to the rules of Cartesian reductionism and probability—or to fundamental processes that need a qualitative interpretation. So the Cartesian positivist bubble has been a permanent epistemological obstacle for critical transformative life sciences.

Critical science constitutes a unique epistemological demand, but it also responds to a reaffirmation of ethics. This is because it requires criticizing data of social and epidemiological inequality and seriously questioning the epistemic or cultural conditions imposed on people, but also denouncing the integrated regressive determination of the material basis of society, with its cultural civilization basis. Critical thinking questions the dominant ideas, practices, and ethos of a particular scientific field.

Broadbent (2013) wrote a book with the suggestive title *Philosophy of Epidemiology*. According to Broadbent, the book answers the question, Why philosophy of epidemiology? When stating why epidemiology is philosophically interesting, Broadbent adduces the following interesting features of "this young science": It focuses on causation; the nonconformity to standard philosophical images of science in experiment and theory; the relative domain insensitivity of its methods; the centrality of its population thinking; and its stakes are high.

Broadbent's (2013) arguments are definitively sharp and useful. We cannot deal with them in-depth here, but some basic comments are mandatory. For reasons provided in Chapter 3, several changes strengthen and place the author's arguments in place with critical science. First, it should not focus restrictively on causation but, rather, on health determination. Second and third, should read some like: epidemiology's nonconformity with lineal Cartesian functional reductionism and the restrictive reductionist experimental logic applied in the social sciences and empiricist theory. Fourth, should not be explained as domain insensitivity but on the contrary, to a careful sensitivity to complex multi-domain objectivity. The fifth argument is agreeable but with the condition that the notion "population" would not refer to an inductive sum of individual observations but to a different essence of the collective phenomena. And the sixth feature is totally correct because epidemiology's stakes are definitively high—as we pretended to demonstrate in chapter 3—but not only for epistemic and moral significance, but on transformative action significance of any science destined to protect and promote human and planetary life.

Serious and well-intentioned researchers operating from the linear Cartesian paradigm are subject to what we call "paradigm bias," which precedes any epidemiological design. All studies of Cartesian facture, even if they use the best design and analysis tools, will be biased.

The Cartesian Bubble: Preliminary Panorama

The Cartesian conception of reality dominates the life sciences. The Cartesian paradigm states that in reality all phenomena are a convergence of parts, and the properties of those parts determine the behavior of the whole. Being the essential elements, those parts preexist and only their conjunction defines the nature and existence of the whole. This operation has been defined as *reduction*, and its methodological matrix is called reductionism (Levins & Lewontin, 1985).

Broadly speaking, the reductionist ontology of Cartesian science, profoundly embedded in functionalist public health and reductionist medicine, can be summarized by the following set of linked operations: *fragmenting* the world into parts or preeminent ontological units (i.e., empirical qualitatively and quantitatively isolated parts of reality); *reifying* those parts as static, fragmented, and individualized elements (i.e., factors, risk factors, and outcomes); associating those parts or ontological fragments by mere *external conjunction; separating* parts from their "contexts and evaluative relations" (i.e., disconnection, decontextualization, and separation); limiting the understanding of movement to the variations of those disconnected parts or *fragmented empirical variables*; and applying the results of those operations to *describe* them, their empirical external connections, and *calculate the probability* of phenomena without explaining their movement and social determination. Later, we discuss why mere lineal causal relations—monocausal or multicausal—are not in themselves a substitute for complex process analysis of the social determination of health. We also reveal its practical political consequences: replacing the encompassing holistic perspective of critical collective health sciences with a narrow focalizing view of functional public health; exchanging the transformative leitmotiv of critical health sciences with a functional scheme of cosmetic public health administrative techniques; substituting the radical perspective of class, gender, and ethnic inequity with a light skirmish for palliatives; and replacing the radical objectives of community-based health action with the technobureaucratic approach of governance (Table 2.1).

Table 2.1 Linear Reductionist and Complex Critical Health Definitions

Functional Linear Thinking	Complex Critical Process Thinking
HEALTH AS OBJECT	
Single plane ("peak of the iceberg") phenomena linearly connected (i.e., reified decontexualized fragments)	Concatenated, multidimensional, and contradictory process movement
Static and fragmented risk factors (i.e., probabilistic entities) causing disease; factorial reality	Process that generates the complex multidimensional movement of collective health, with embodiments in particular class/gender/ethnic and individual conditions
THE SUBJECT OF HEALTH	
Lineal, one-plane vision	Explaining concatenated, contextualized complex multidimensional movement
One discipline biomedical vision	Thinking transdisciplinarily: not simple juxtaposition of knowledges and their complementarity but mutual transvaluation (*Oxford Encyclopedia*)
Monocultural vision, centered in positivist academic monism	Intercultural knowledge building and transevaluation
Conception of reality centered on logical empiricism and systems theory (structural functionalism)	Meta-critical dialectic thinking (i.e., integrating the different critical epistemologies to transform reality: criticism of accumulation, functionalist instrumental reason, and uncritical subjectivity)

(continued)

Table 2.1 **Continued**

Functional Linear Thinking	Complex Critical Process Thinking
THE CONCEPTION OF PRAXIS	
Focalized risk factors action, with their systematization based on empirical differences and probabilistic weight	Characterizing action as meta-critical counteractive movement, sensitive reasoning, multidimensional neohumanism; operation on contradictions of critical processes, based on a radical notion of inequity and the analysis of strategic interests of the common good

The logic we have just described, reinforced by influential bio-medical determinism, when applied within public administration produces the divorce of health indicators from their social and cultural contexts. When considered for administrative and planning purposes, epidemiologic reasoning operates under the premise that a discretional inventory of health standard indices alone will suffice as an evaluatory tool for assessing the success of social policies. Some classical indicators of changes in morbidity and mortality rates, or the degree of health services coverage, are considered, in themselves, to be the gold standard for weighing the effectiveness of public policy and governance. Such evaluations are therefore often limited to the analysis of isolated programs and services provision and to classical epidemiological indicators. From this perspective, when a society goes from "bad rates" to "less bad rates," the illusion of success is declared.

Qualitative research is also affected by Cartesian bias. It has been developed to account for numerical reductionism to complement the scientific method. It "relies on text and image data, has unique steps in data analysis, and draws on diverse designs" (Aspin, 1995, p. 21). Some methodologists recognize the following as its principal strengths: collecting data directly in the field; direct data collection by researchers who analyze documents, observe conduct, or interview informants; relying on multiple data sources; including important deductive moments to build patterns, categories, and themes; keeping a focus on meanings defined by participants; maintaining an emergent, constantly developing design; researcher reflexivity and self-consciousness; and a holistic account of the problem (Creswell, 2014). But it is also true that different theories have influenced the paradigm-driven development of qualitative research—that is, positivism, critical theory, constructivism, phenomenology, symbolic interactionism, and grounded theory (Punch, 2016). The latter has been most influential, and according to Creswell (2014) can be explained as follows: "The researcher derives a general, abstract theory of a process, action, or interaction grounded in the views of participants . . . using multiple stages of data collection and the refinement and interrelationship of categories of information" (p. 14). This form of qualitative inductivism also occurs in Cartesian reductionism.

In Chapter 3, we discuss how Cartesian empiricism as a strategic cog of hegemonic science not only imposes the positivist ontology or qualitative cultural relativism we have just summarized but also, most important, constrains the philosophical stance of the life and health sciences within an anthropocentric individualist functional framework.

Social Determination of Health: Overcoming the Illusions of Linear Causality

As we have repeatedly argued in previous sections, the cardinal challenge of critical theory/method is to overcome the lineal single-plane causality of conventional epidemiology by super-seding the reductionist inductive chain we have explained and that is applied in the Cartesian *principle of correspondence* (Figure 2.1).

The knowledge illusion of linear reductionist tip-of-the-iceberg-type thinking resides in substituting the explanation of a complex multidimensional movement with mere description and prediction of partial variations and correlations. The knowledge illusion also resides in mistaking the sophistication of empirical descriptions—either qualitative or quantitative—for the under-standing of complex movement that explains those empirical

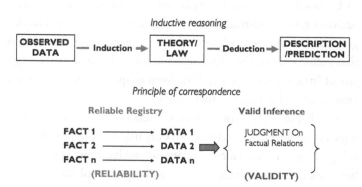

Figure 2.1 The principle of correspondence and empirical induction.

expressions. Instead of understanding the processes that explain epidemiological determination, it applies firsthand perceptions to *describe* factual variations and their empirical external connections and to *calculate the probability* of such phenomena. In other words, it describes variables and their external variations without explaining the complex social determination of health.

Complexity and Critical Science

When taking a scientific position on health as a complex dynamic process, we invariably need to put forward a consistent argument regarding *complexity*. Different perspectives converge to provide a critical outlook of this social feature. They all disprove the conceptual and methodological implications of the positivist linear single plane perspective. A crucial contemporary discussion about health as a complex process is fundamental in redefining the study object of epidemiology.

First, the idea that health is an object that takes its form within the inherent dynamic articulation of diverse types of phenomena, therefore demanding a *transdisciplinarity* approach, is one important element of complex thinking. As Morin (201) explains in his view of complexity,

> We are at the same time biological, social, cultural, psychic and spiritual beings, it is evident that complexity is what attempts to conceive the articulation, identity, and difference of all these aspects. . . . In fact the aspiration of complexity tends towards multidimensional knowledge. (pp. 176–177; translated by the author).

From this perspective, one would clearly agree that critical epidemiology necessarily requires a complex transdisciplinary approach. This argument also leads to the broader notion of intercultural knowledge.

Second, in building a complex thinking approach to health, it is crucial to reexamine the different degrees of complexity that characterize processes pertaining to the various dimensions of reality that constitute health's *multidimensionality*. This characteristic involves understanding our social–epidemiological reality as a dynamic interrelated movement of three different domains: the general (G) domain of society (i.e., social reproduction and broader nature–society environmental metabolic relations); the typical particular (P) and collective *modes of living* of socially determined groups subject to social and specific metabolic relations (i.e., social class, gender, and ethnocultural power and metabolic relations) and the individual (I) domain of persons/families with their specific personal *styles of living*[7] and corporal psychological embodiments (i.e., phenotypic, genotypic, psychological, and spiritual).

The permanent evolution of those different domains is not essentially independent, as complex movement is not a simple sum of adjacent parts. There is dialectic interplay between the unifying trend of the reproduction of society as a whole and the diversifying movement generated due to the relative autonomy of parts that press to maintain their diversity. This determining interplay

---

7. Here, as we further explain later, it is very important to distinguish our notion of *styles of living* with the conventional English concept of "lifestyles." It is also important to differentiate it from our notion of collective *modes of living*.

accounts for the *dialectic movement* of complex reality, in which the reproduction of *unity* is counteracted by the reproduction of *diversity*. In sociological terms, this involves the relation between collective and individual social reproduction, a movement that is crucial for understanding the genesis of health conditions. Juan Samaja (1997) appropriately described its integral nature by maintaining in his analysis the two contradictory trends: on the one hand, a creative process that arises from the particular domain—and even from the individuals—pushing to transform the general terms of reproduction and increase diversity and, on the other hand, a counteractive movement on the part of broader society to reproduce its general existence. This clarification was very important for the debate within social sciences and epidemiology because it gave a new sense of direction to the discussion about personal versus collective rule in society. We now better understand that both are permanently active as dynamic sources of social movement. Health correspondingly depends on the wider process of social determination; notwithstanding, the relative autonomy of individual action also accounts for important modifications.

This oppositional development of *unity (integration) versus diversity* of health as a whole and health as a particular and individual process also entails a double epistemological (interpretative)—methodological challenge: (1) to eliminate the false separations of Cartesian logic and (2) to correct the empiricist conception of multidimensionality.

One major challenge is to apply an epistemological paradigm that retains the cognitive dialectic of categories that positivist science has separated. In fact, positivist logic established a set of false separations that were utilized to subordinate scientific interpretations to its empiricist rules of objectivity (i.e., the notions of matter, motion, and number). This separation was first applied in astronomy and physics and later in physiology and biology (Irvine, Miles, & Evans, 1979, p. 66). Irvine et al. highlight some cases of uncoupling that distorted scientific thinking:

Subject	Object
Purpose	Mechanism
Value	Fact
Internal	External
Secondary	Primary (properties)
Thought	Extension
Mind	Body
Culture	Nature
Society	Science

The concepts in the first column were replaced by the concepts in the second column. This completely changed the interpretative essence of reality. The broader cognitive categories of the first column were reduced to the more descriptive and partial elements of the second column (Irvine et al., 1979, p. 66), and this reduction converted reality into a single-plane empirical world (Figure 2.2).

This type of cognition had important consequences for conventional epidemiological positivist methodology. From the specific concerns of critical epidemiology, we must recognize seven

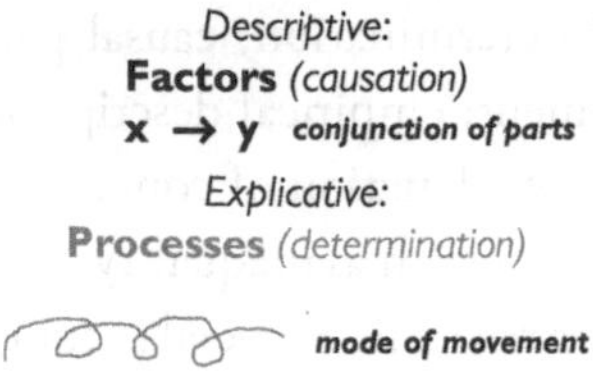

Descriptive:
Factors *(causation)*
x → y *conjunction of parts*
Explicative:
Processes *(determination)*

mode of movement

Figure 2.2 The two visions: factors that describe conjunctions versus processes that explain movement.

other conceptual substitutions appropriate to a linear functional description of health:

Collective	Individual
Processes	Factors
Subsumption	Conjunction
Determination	Causality (i.e., causes or determinants)
Embodiment	Causal pathogenicity
Explanation	Description, prediction
Inequity	Inequality, difference

The cognitive and logic implications of these substitutions are discussed in relation to the methodological breaks that we detail later. At this point, it is necessary to recognize that conventional public health and Cartesian epidemiological reasoning have applied many of those substitutions in order to subordinate their logic to the empiricist rules of objectivity: the individual (part) instead of the collective; causal risk factors instead of determining processes; linear conjunction instead of dialectic subsumption;

causality instead of determination; causal pathogenicity instead of dialectic embodiment; empirical description and probabilistic prediction instead of explanation of complex determination; and phenomenal expressions such as inequality or difference instead of the underlying power relations of social inequity.

A second important undertaking is to recover the unity and interdependence that exists in multidimensional reality as a result of the ontological connection between processes that pertain to different dimensions. This is of paramount importance to health studies. It entails the task of restating the relations that define health and their manifold movement. Deciphering the essence and factual evidence of such connections between the general (G), particular (P), and individual (I) processes is precisely the main challenge of critical epidemiology, which is to grasp the essence of health as a socially determined multidimensional movement. This is what we aimed at when we incorporated the notion of social determination of health into our interpretative model in order to expand the empirical causal view, based on the firsthand, formal conjunction of "independent," "dependent," and "intervening" empirically defined variables—in other words, the notion of variables taken as fragmented expressions or segments, detached from their respective domains of reality and subject to mere external connection. Later, we discuss our methodology for assuming variables as nodal expressions of a broader movement and its critical processes.

The social determination of health process is complex not only because of its multidimensional nature but also because the dynamicity of its health conditioning process encompasses the contradictory movement of both concrete healthy, life-supportive, protecting subprocesses and concrete unhealthy, harmful, and destructive subprocesses. As explained previously, this multidimensional movement develops simultaneously and interdependently in all three dimensions (G/P/I); in all three domains, there are different contradictions between protective and destructive health processes.

As discussed previously, the social determination movement and its health-related aspects develop according to the broader structured characteristics and power relations of a defined social formation [i.e., social relations, modes of social reproduction (wealth production and accumulation), and metabolism with nature] and typical collective modes of living of socially determined groups subject to social relations (i.e., class position intertwined with gender and ethnic sociocultural relations)—all of which define their health equity status or potential—and, finally, in the individual (I) domain of persons/families with their specific personal styles of living and corporal psychological embodiments (i.e., phenotype, genotype, mind, and spiritual) (Figure 2.3).

By this point, some readers may have asked themselves, What is so important about understanding and making clear the multidimensional unity and the contradictory protective–destructive nature of health? The straightforward answer is because it is indispensable to discover the essence of the health production and distribution process that epidemiology needs to reveal. And also because in order to comply with Virchow's (1848) ethical demand for radical measures and not palliatives—in order to get into real, consistent, and profound health promotion and prevention—we must reconnect what functionalist science disconnected and penetrate into the destructive nature of the economic system and its alienating civilization.

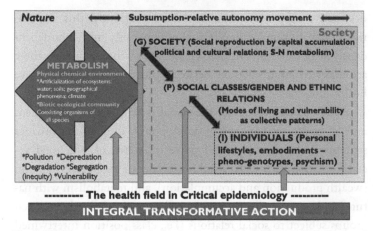

Figure 2.3 The social determination of health (complex—multidimensional movement) (Breilh, 1977, 2003a, 2015a). G, general; I, individual; P, particular.

Breilh, J. (2015a). Epidemiología crítica latinoamericana: Raíces, desarrollos recientes y ruptura metodológica. In *Tras las huellas de la determinación* (Memorias de Seminario Inter-universitario de determinación social de la salud; pp. 19–75). Bogotá, Columbia: Universidad Nacional de Colombia.

A personal experience I want to share with readers is relevant to the arguments presented in this section. I met Nancy Krieger for the first time in Quito, Ecuador, when she attended an international seminar in the 1980s that was organized to debate critical epidemiology and social *determination* of health. Researchers from 12 countries were convoked to share and discuss our challenges and contributions. Many years later, Krieger and I teamed up again on the same side of the international critical transformative epidemiological science debate. Two roundtables were held—one part of the World Conference on Social Determinants of Health, organized by WHO (Rio de Janeiro, 2011), and another in the 8th International Seminar on Public Health, planned by the National University of Colombia (Bogotá, 2013) to focus on "social determination of health" as theory for the 21st century. In both cases, our theoretical stances were complementary. Here, what is relevant to highlight is Krieger's important contribution in positioning the notion of *embodiment* (Krieger, 2005, 2013). From the perspective of my work, it entailed a perfect and necessary fit for my theory on social determination and my proposed substitution of conjunctive causality with determination by subsumption. Later, I expand this argument.

Social Determination: Social Reproduction, Metabolism, Subsumption/Embodiment, and Inequity

Determination is no doubt the cardinal category of critical epidemiology in relation to its understanding of the production and distribution of health, just as *causality* is the central notion of Cartesian linear empiricist epidemiology.

The philosophical fundaments of conventional linear causality can be traced back to the empiricist works of Locke and Berkeley and, most important, to David Hume's *Treatise of Human Nature* (1740/1967). In this influential work, the Scottish philosopher states the principles of association (i.e., resemblance, contiguity, and causation) that became the pillars of his Aristotelian conception of scientific knowledge as the revealing of causes and causal inference. Austin Bradford Hill (1965) developed his criteria for determining a causal association, whereas emblematic epidemiologists such as Brian McMahon (1975) with his "web of causation" and Kenneth Rothman and Timothy Greenland

(1998) with their constellation of causes explicitly assume causal reasoning as the cardinal element of their important scientific work. Mainstream positivist health science consequently operates under the premise that causality constitutes what has been critically defined as the big organizing rationality of the Universe (Rorty, 1994).

The problem we face, leaving aside the valuable contributions and technical advancements of causal epidemiology, is that reductionism hinders the sophisticated potentialities of many of its own achievements. Causal reasoning entails a succession of reductions of Cartesian science, brilliantly explained by Bhaskar (1986), that operate along empirical lines. I have summarized this extremely important clarification as follows (Breilh, 2003a):

Once only empirical reality is included as patterns of events, excluding the other domains (that is, excluding the generative processes and the current non-empirical processes), it proceeds to incorporate from those patterns only those that are constant conjunctions (which means the empirical processes associated stably as variables), leaving out the constant non-associative movement patterns (i.e. the variables that did not yield significant correlations); finally, of those constant conjunctions establishes an "experiment," or better in the case of epidemiology, a "proxy" as a closed system. Thus the inductive empirical knowledge begins to close its logical cycle and establishes the causal conclusion:

Demonstrated constant conjunction = causal law = knowledge
Hence also its practical logic follows:

Application = instrumental success = system functionality
(p. 34)

Here, the core problem is reducing our complex world to demonstrated constant conjunctions detached from their profound determining connections through an experimental logic.

So in order to develop an alternative epidemiological rationale, while at the same time retaining the valid contributions and experience of the past, it was imperative to break the reductionist mold, proposing an interpretative substitute for causality. We needed a new paradigm that would give us back the vision of reality as movement, as ongoing processes and not stationary factors. A shift was required in order to reconnect the parts of that fragmented reality within a real integrative multidimensionality, to health's complexity in the contradiction of the protective and harmful processes and, as a consequence, to not only describe the empirical phenomena and make predictions but also explain the health process in an integral way. Only then could epidemiology be labeled a penetrating, transformative, and emancipating discipline.

Because the alternative theoretical framework needed to explain the production and distribution of health, we chose five categories as fundamental cognitive elements: determination, natural and social reproduction, society–nature metabolism, subsumption[8], and inequity. These categories respectively explain: the movement; the overall articulating logic of that movement; the

---

8. *Subsumption* is a notion we applied in epidemiology that we connect to the category *embodiment* proposed by Nancy Krieger.

determining weight of the ecosystem; the social-biological relation; and the growing health gap that forms part of health's complexity in our societies. In other words, these provide a new vision that allows us to avoid the divisions and substitutions of the empiricist logic we are questioning. We now examine this challenge in more detail.

The dialectic explanation of movement and connection that causality does not allow requires overcoming causal notions. The transformation of reality that yields health consequences cannot reside solely in causal relations. We therefore had to work for a number of years in order to find a better system for explaining the complexity of the epidemiological movement. If reality moves not just by means of causal relations, we had to understand the alternative complete interpretative model that would allow us to explain health-generating processes. If epidemiological movement is not limited to quantitative variations (mechanism), if it is not reduced to an external causal production, and if variation is not reduced to a unique conjunction relationship, then we needed to develop a different approach that entailed answering a different question: How do we explain epidemiological movement as a complex determining phenomenon?

In his valuable book *The Principle of Causality in Modern Science*, Mario Bunge (1972) argues that the facts which govern life are determined, not only caused. In searching for an alternative category that would encompass more than the notion of causality, he explored the category of *determination*. He found that it had three scientific meanings: (1) the property or attribute of things that have defined characteristics; (2) the necessary and unique connection between things, events, states, and qualities (causal, not generative or productive link); and (3) a mode of becoming—how a process becomes such and acquires its characteristics.

The third meaning, corresponding to the form (act or process) by which an object acquires its properties, precisely resolved our epistemological requirement. In this way, we came to understand that epidemiological processes not only have empirically defined characteristics, which can be observed and recorded as variables, but also acquire them in defined forms or processes that transcend causal links because they explain movement and generative power that go beyond causal conjunctions. The scope of epidemiological observation, then, is not limited to the phenomenon (i.e., single-plane "tip of the iceberg") but must encompass the underlying determinant movements that generate the empirically observable elements. That is because epidemiological processes operate in a multidimensional social–natural context that determines their contents and scale. They extend their roots in all three dimensions (G/P/I) with their specific social relations, spaces, and territories. Those relations constitute the determining mold or material basis of social determination. At the same time, the political, cultural, and spiritual relations and conditions that make up a part of social reproduction intervene in the building and transformation of the social determination processes.

A complex, fascinating dialectic defines and explains, through concrete forms of movement in each of the dimensions of reality,(1) how epidemiological processes become such and acquire their characteristics and (2) the observable embodiments of which empirical qualitative and quantitative phenomena form part. This finding became a major turning point in our work and opened doors to new challenges. Later, we further explain determination and illustrate this reasoning with a concrete example.

In its complexity, epidemiological movement encompasses natural organic and inorganic processes as well as social processes. But nonsocial and social processes are determined differently: The former basically operate under their own chemical or biological and instinctive conditionings (of course subsumed in social conditions), whereas social movement is determined by historical projects consciously defined by human collectives. This was explained this in a Pan American Health Organization/WHO publication as a dialectical subsumption relations system, among domains of different complexity (Breilh, 1994). This difference has been explained by Georg Lukács (2013) as a teleological[9] problem. In his ontology, he differentiated the inorganic and organic domains from the social by considering the former as nonpurposeful, whereas the social domain would be teleological in the sense of conscious design of purpose.

Our previous argument and the understanding of the relation between the social and environmental–biological processes require a clear understanding of the difference between *natural reproduction* and social reproduction. Preconscious animal reproduction operates by making transformations in nature in order to produce elements that allow animals to obtain their means of survival (food, warmth, rest, play, etc.). They manage this movement in response to a natural instinct that operates as a determinant biological norm in the absence of conscious purposeful drive. This

---

9. Teleological: exhibiting or relating to design or purpose (*Merriam-Webster Dictionary*: https://www.merriam-webster.com/dictionary/teleological#other-words).

natural order functions without language, without representation of the "other," and without conscious purposefulness. That is, animal processes in themselves lack historic determination. Animals need by instinct, they communicate with each other through signs, and their biological capacities can reach amazing levels of performance and allow for almost "perfect" instinct-driven solutions. Nonetheless, in the case of bees, for example, the difference between their perfectly built hives and the imperfect or even clumsy construction of a house by an unskilled human is the fact that the former was produced instinctively, without preconceived purpose, whereas the imperfect house was the purposeful product of a conscious project.

However, at this point we must emphasize the eco-epidemiological importance of the consequences of social production in the process of nature's artificialization—that is, the social determination of ecosystem health. Although animal life functions according to the rules of instinct and a primitive psychic system, the fact that animals' natural reproduction, life cycles, and breeding modes, as well as territorial habitats, are permanently transformed by the social–natural metabolism and subject to forms of artificialization carries with it the most destructive consequences. Influenced by critical epidemiology, a new zoonotic disease model has been developing as part of a different animal health paradigm (Acero, 2010). The quintessence of negative, massive transformation of animal life can be observed in the social–natural spaces of extractivism, either because extractive-derived hazards (agricultural pesticides, heavy metals from mining, etc.) kill many animals and in many cases affect their ecological role—for example, poisoning pollinizing bees that sustain vegetable reproduction—or because large-scale business concentrates immense numbers of animals in gigantic industrial breeding farms (poultry, swine, etc.). The profit-geared design and operation of these farms is therefore permanently affecting the territorial health of large regions, destroying or severely affecting the rights of natural life beings, and dramatically increasing the contamination of regional soils and water systems. The Johns Hopkins University Pew Commission on Industrial Farm Animal Production (2008, p. 35) fully documented the devastating impacts of corporate animal farms in four primary areas: public health, the environment, animal welfare, and rural communities. It demonstrated how the shift from the innocuous family farm system to highly concentrated profit-oriented business systems is provoking an array of human, animal, and general ecosystem effects. The global implantation of high-tech, nature-unfriendly, insensible megafarms not only has expanded an increasingly unfair agricultural system but also has caused destructive embodiments in animals, inducing abnormalities in their physiology; causing uncontrolled damage through genetic modifications and reproductive organ anomalies; transforming their health by streamlining the process of raising animals for profit, including standardized feed for rapid weight gain and uniformity; and through genetic operations. All this artificialization is implemented for rapid profit and capital accumulation. These megafarms are also contributing to the increase in the pool of antibiotic-resistant bacteria due to the overuse of antibiotics; to air quality problems; to the contamination of rivers, streams, and coastal waters with concentrated animal waste; to animal welfare problems, mainly as a result of the extremely close quarters in which the animals are housed; and to significant shifts in the social structure and economy of many farming regions throughout the country. Here, we have a colossal embodiment of deleterious mechanisms within global and local ecosystems. This expanded concept of embodiment is defined later.

We launched our first version of a dialectical determination in the late 1970s (Breilh, 1977) through a systematic critique of McMahon's (1975) causal web theory and of the ecosystem model based on the Parsonian[10] systems theory of the "natural history of disease" (Leavell & Clark, 1965). We shifted the logic of determination:

> Causal *factors* or "determinants" that describe or predict, to Generative *processes* that operate through intrinsic connections between distinct domains that explain the forms of movement that engender transformations.

Here, again, to comprehend health as movement, we had to embed its analysis in the transforming process of social reproduction. The challenge was to understand the material core and the domains of social transformations (see Figure 2.3). Doing so implied deciphering the dynamic development of modes of production and consumption, which take different social forms according to the strategic interests governing society. Notwithstanding the fact that the mode of social reproduction has changed throughout history, since the initiation of capitalist modernity it has taken the

---

10. Talcott Parson's "systems theory," the so-called *structural functionalism*, proclaimed reality as a system composed of a set of systems that permanently tend toward equilibrium, adaptation, and adjustment in order to attain certain functional roles (Parsons, 1991).

form of capital accumulation.[11] But social reproduction does not only encompass a material core but also simultaneously involves a conscious, historical, cultural creation process; it also entails certain power relations and forms of political organization and, most important, the metabolic relations of society with nature that we have outlined.

By means of all these integrated processes, capital accumulation has become the fundamental general matrix not only for reproducing the social, social–environmental, and human social–biological processes of our market societies but also of particular modes of living and ever-growing health inequity that subordinate social classes—traversed by gender and ethnocultural asymmetries/experience. Capital accumulation superimposes itself on the logic, trends, and hegemonic characteristics of all spaces and territories. It binds the historically unequal access to human and social rights to a power-based distribution of rent and income. By doing so, it conditions and puts limits on the degree of economic, political, and cultural power that conflicting social groups can acquire, as well as on the corresponding political disputes and alliances that characterize their relations. The capital accumulation matrix determines ecosystem relations in every sector of social space and the environmental contrasts that inequity generates

11. *Capital accumulation* at its core results from the surplus value that any production company generates by extracting from the productive cycle of workers additional value to that of the labor force measured by the same unit of time. If the labor force generates per day or per hour a value greater than the value of its salary for that period, surplus capital is generated. Nonetheless, there are other sources of cyclic accumulation involved that we explain in this chapter.

in distinct territories and neighborhoods. All these congruent movements for guaranteeing the reproduction of capital do not operate separately; their movement is interdependent. What provides the overall congruency of the general social reproduction of accumulation is the process of subsumption, as we discuss later.

Geographical spaces and their ecosystems encompass concrete territorial forms of social reproduction. They are a product of the mode of social reproduction and its ways of transforming social space and nature, but concomitantly they actively contribute to its transformation. This *metabolism* of society and nature cuts across all dimensions of the process of the social determination of health and traverses all social–natural subsumption processes. Karl Marx first enounced the economical–political definition of a metabolic movement in his transcendental work on political economy (Marx, 1981). He referred to the processes between socially organized humans and nature where, through their own actions, they mediate, regulate and determine their metabolism with nature. By doing so, he linked his critical realist vision of both society and nature, thus providing a most potent explanation of critical ecology (Foster, 2000). In this abridged account, this dialectic concept surpasses *empirical ecology* theories—which have applied reductionist so-called ecosystem health paradigms—instead of explaining the social historical determination and territoriality of the relations between Nature and Society. At the same time, these relations make part of the healthy–unhealthy dynamics of such metabolism. Society–nature metabolism implies subprocesses of utilization, transformation, distribution, consumption, and excretion, which occur in all three dimensions (G/P/I), becoming a crucial element of social life and one crucial environmental embodiment of historical development. Unfortunately, society's dominant productive apparatus systematically provokes a large-scale inappropriate artificialization of nature's biocenosis (i.e., biotic or ecological communities; organisms of all species that co-exist) and shapes its biotope (i.e., the physical and chemical setting and environmental conditions that operate as the vital space of flora and fauna), and it does so in ways that multiply unhealthy ecosystems.

As we have insisted, social reproduction operates in all three domains (G/P/I), but in each domain its movement involves different levels of complexity, ranging from the major influence of the general processes to the impact of less convoluted individual processes. In that complex reproductive movement, the weightier, more complex *general* domain processes subsume the *particular* less intricate processes and, at the same time, these subsume the lesser influence of the less convoluted *individual* processes. In Chapter 3, we touch again on the importance of *subsumption*, but for now we only state that it explains the inherent determining connection of processes pertaining to different domains of complexity of social reproduction, where the more intricate subsystem imposes its conditions on the movement of the least complex. The less complex individual biopsychological movement in people develops with its own psychological, physiological, and genetic natural reproduction rules, but their complete operation corresponds with and is influenced by the conditions of social reproduction. We now illustrate this crucial argument.

It is well known that autism, for instance, as with obesity and other pandemic problems, shows a rapid increase in global incidence and prevalence. Here again, different conflicting paradigms provide radically diverse epidemiological insights. The dominant vision unfortunately comes from an empiricist biomedical and conventional functional public health perspective. Fortunately, there is a growing awareness about the urgency of a paradigm shift in order to deal with 21st-century children's health from a critical social epidemiological perspective. For instance, groundbreaking approaches are focusing on the complex relations between neurodevelopmental disabilities, including autism, attention-deficit/hyperactivity disorder, and dyslexia, and other cognitive impairments that are more frequently diagnosed and related to wide systematic exposure to industrial chemicals that injure the developing brain (Grandjean & Landrigan, 2014). It is a cardinal problem for vulnerable communities upset by typical class-related vulnerabilities to neurobehavioral impacts of environmental toxicity. Early life exposures to neurotoxic chemicals affect children's developmental programming and functional maturation, provoking neurological degenerative changes. More than 5,000 children's products, such as clothing, toys, and shoes, have been recognized in certain regions as containing any of 66 chemicals of high risk to children, including toxic metals such as cadmium, mercury, cobalt, antimony, and molybdenum, and organic compounds such as methyl ethyl ketone and ethylene glycol, as well as phthalates (Uding & Schreder, 2015).

As mentioned previously, the powerful notion of embodiment, proposed by Krieger (2011) and used in the sense of giving a concrete perceptible form or body to a process, is integrated in our theoretical framework with the notion of subsumption. We can also expand this powerful category of Krieger's important interpretative tool of social–biological relation to other sorts of incarnations (metaphorically speaking) that are generated in different domains. Subsumption involves the conditioning of a less complex movement by a more complex one. For example, the movement of capital accumulation (general dimension G) subsumes that of particular modes of living (particular dimension P); at the same time, these subsume individual styles of living (individual dimension I), and this movement concomitantly conditions the phenotypic, genotypic, and psychological processes of an individual. Subsumption is not a unidirectional mechanical relationship but, rather, a dialectic movement that is counteracted due to the relative autonomy and generative potentiality of less complex processes. On the other hand, the transitive verb *embodying* means "to give a body to," "to make concrete and perceptible," and "to cause to become a body."[12] As stated previously, we have extended the notion "to make concrete and perceptible" to the social or collective domain. This was indispensable not only because the human being experiences embodiments or incarnations of an epidemiologically generating process but also because, as we illustrate in the case of the social determination of vector-borne diseases in an agro-industrial territory, the movement produces social, geophysical–ecosystem, or collective human embodiments that we use methodologically to explain and situate certain specific variations (i.e., socially rather than probabilistically defined variables) and structure our different approach according to qualitative and quantitative research (Figure 2.4).

---

12. *Merriam-Webster Dictionary* (https://www.merriam-webster.com/dictionary/embodying).

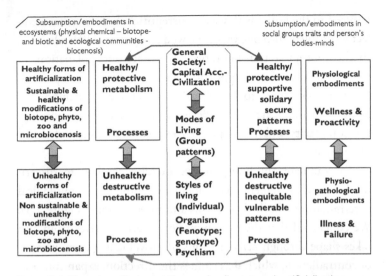

Figure 2.4 Domains of subsumption, embodiment, and artificialization.

Breilh, J. (1977). Crítica a la interpretación ecológico funcionalista de la epidemiología: Un ensayo de desmitificación del proceso salud enfermedad. Mexico City, Mexico: Universidad Autónoma Metropolitana de Xochimilco.

It is important to note that Cartesian lineal epidemiology, in consonance with its positivist rules of objectivity, assumes individual phenomena as the central reference, surrounded externally by so-called social variables or risk factors. The conceptual and methodological flaws of this viewpoint are discussed later, but for now it is necessary to bring the reader's attention to the ostensible extremely negative consequence of victim blaming, which results from separating individual conditions from their collective determining processes. As in the case of the obesity pandemic mentioned in the Introduction, when our scope of interpretation is reduced to the individual, we are surreptitiously converting a collective problem into one that is viewed as a personal lifestyle issue. By this conceptual transfiguration, we reduce our explanations to individual "causes" and apportion the entire blame for epidemiological occurrences to individuals and families. An important break with this Cartesian logic is the recovery of the ontological complexity and interdependence of collective and individual phenomena.

To complete our interpretative exercise, we had to discern the forms of movement that concur in complex epidemiological determination—both their forms and interrelations (Figure 2.5). We concluded that the determination process derives from and takes shape through certain forms of movement: (1) movement of contradiction, which determines the direction, expansion, and intensity of the movement of less complex processes with their conditions of subsumption and corresponding embodiments; (2) causal movement, which determines the forms of cause–effect efficient conjunctions; (3) feedback movement, which determines the capacity of adaptive–transformative system regulation; (4) probabilistic movement, which determines the random

- **Movement of contradictions**
  (determines direction and intensity of
  less complex processes – conditions subsumption)
- **Causality**
- **Feedback**
- **Probabilistic**
- Uncertain movement **("fuzzy") and chaotic**

Figure 2.5 Components of the social determination movement (mode of becoming and acquiring characteristics).

variation of regular systems under determined degrees of freedom; and (5) uncertain movement ("fuzzy") in complex quality quantifier systems with high, formal, nonlineal complexity and chaotic movement of irregular system processes. These different forms of movement can be modeled and analyzed using different mathematical tools. Unlike linear Cartesian epidemiology, in critical epidemiology the process of data collection and analysis of each form of movement will be subjected to the dimensions of determination (G/P/I)—their dialectical relations of subsumption and relative autonomy. Specifically, this analysis uses variables but is not based on them; rather, it is based on critical processes that allow for the explanation of these modes of movement.

At this point, after discussing the flaws and implications of causal thinking in epidemiology, we need to call the attention of our readers to the crucial need to differentiate the category of social *determination* of health that we are putting forward as antithetical to causal philosophy from the notion of the social *determinants* of health that constitutes a cardinal concept of the dominant epidemiological and public health narratives and, unfortunately, of some expressions of conventional epidemiology that are considered progressive.

Social Determinants or Social Determination: Institutional Reformism or Radical Reform

The Commission on Social Determinants of Health was established by WHO in March 2005 "to support countries and global health partners in addressing the social factors leading to ill health and health inequities" (WHO, 2019). Within well-informed progressive academic scenarios of the South, at first glance this "new" commission's title incited a feeling of hope. The announcement was made after three long decades of difficult creative battles on the part of Latin American researchers, and corresponding ground-breaking publications in Spanish and Portuguese. At this point, we thought voices of the South were starting to be taken into consideration; the important academic profiles of the commission's members constituted a promissory signal.

Unfortunately, this was not the case, and with time we understood that, willingly or not, science from the Global South was not considered. What was at stake then, and even more now, was the real emancipatory essence of the new paradigm. The social determination paradigm is a commitment to a new public and collective health philosophy. Consequently, we have proclaimed in different international forums the importance of a democratic, mind-opening debate on the fundamentals of critical epidemiology as a tool for health policy and planning; it is an irreplaceable instrument to discern the best direction to take at the crossroads between health *reformism* and health *reform*. The former means changing some forms (i.e., "causes" or "factors") so that the social substance is sustained, whereas reform means making changes that compete with the existing substance in order to open up the entire system to change (Echeverría, 1990). It entails forms of collective, transformative practice linked to the strategic interests of the affected communities and aware citizens, who need to change structural health inequity and correspondingly organize a new form of public health.

Thus, in order to carry out a thorough examination of the theoretical pillars and political guidelines of the "determinants" theory, our movement organized three scientific meetings, and the publication of their respective records, in Brazil (Passos Nogueira, 2010), Mexico (Eibenschutz, Tamez, & González, 2011), and Colombia (Morales & Eslava, 2015). Unfortunately, our collective, critical conclusion about the determinants theory was disenchanting. Aside from the good intentions underlying the social "determinants" of health paradigm—as defined by its principal members and mentors (Marmot & Wilkinson, 2006)—in practice it implied a relapse into linear empiricist causality and amounted to a refreshed functionalist health governance scheme. It is important to note that at the beginning of our work in the late 1970s, we proposed the epidemiological use of the concept *determination*. More than 30 years later, when the concept *determinants* was first used epidemiologically, we were not totally clear, as is now the case, about the vital nuances of this semantic difference. But with time, our efforts demonstrated the difference. What is now evident is that the neocausal paradigm of determinants had superimposed some of the original categories that Latin American authors had used and publicized widely, while inserting them in the same empiricist–functional mold (Table 2.2).

Looking at this matter objectively, it was surprising that beyond the good intentions of WHO in conforming regional subcommissions and integrating some scholars from the Global South, the consistent and by then pioneering amply circulated bibliography published by Latin American scientists was not even mentioned, let alone incorporated into the discussions about a new epidemiology. Many years before the commission was convened, we had worked, both conceptually and practically, to develop our social determination philosophy, construct

Table 2.2 Contrasting Paradigms: Social Determination and Social Determinants (Three Dimensions of Epistemological Description)

Epistemological Dimension	Social Determinants of Health	Social Determination of Health
Health as an object	Determinants as causes of a causal constellation ("causes of the causes") Causes in a web of causal conjunction	Determination as a multidimensional movement; connection among dimensions of reality: general (G), particular (P), and individual (I) Processes articulated to the social relations of society
Health as a cognitive subject	Reformist institutional perspective Vision from policies and values for redistributive governance Technical critique from the public servants'/ decision-makers' perspective	Collective community-based perspective of reform from a social health system transformative struggle Critique of market civilizations Radical critical subject from the social transformation perspective Social empowered participation and the right of accountable public social alliance

Table 2.2 Continued

Epistemological Dimension	Social Determinants of Health	Social Determination of Health
Health as praxis/ agency	Institutional policies and practice for redistributive governance, in the framework of system sustainability Agency against social factors (causes) that impede or limit redistributive governance	Social intercultural practice as historical movement, linked to strategic interests of subjugated class–gender– ethnic groups Struggle for radical transformation that encompasses inequitable social relations; unhealthy modes of living and alienating cultural patterns; unhealthy territories and metabolisms; empowerment of subjugated social, gender, and ethnic groups

Based on Breilh, J. (2003a). *Epidemiología crítica ciencia emancipadora e interculturalidad*. Buenos Aires, Argentina: Lugar Editoral; and Breilh, J. (2015a). Epidemiología crítica: Raíces, desarrollos recientes y ruptura metodológica. In C. Morales & J. C. Eslava (Eds.), *Tras las huellas de la determinación* (pp. 19–75). Bogotá, Colombia: Universidad Nacional.

a pioneering theory, renew methodology, and generate bold action programs. Latin American critical epidemiology had become a consistent facet of our continental movement of social medicine. By then, our bibliography was clearly familiar to progressive scholars of the North who published important reviews in high-impact English journals (Waitzkin, Iriart, Estrada, & Lamadrid, 2001). However, these advanced scientific contributions and proposals from the South were bluntly ignored by the proponents of new materials from the North, in their Eurocentric spirit.

Willingly or not, from our perspective, a form of epistemicide has taken place. However, for the benefit of a radical paradigm on health equality and environmental justice, we need to consolidate the emancipatory consequences that spring from this important 21st-century controversy between the Latin American paradigm and the functional logic of the "determinants" approach that operates in the linear fragmenting logic of causalism (i.e., "causes of the causes"), cherishing redistributive governance over "factors" as its leitmotiv. We need to bring this important discussion to academic and institutional scenarios if we want to overcome the conservative cosmetic functionalist strategy that has been enthroned among public servants and important university departments. The current global health crisis demands a new understanding and form of governance that decolonizes international scientific and technical cooperation and builds new democratic, respectful, and intercultural ties between the North and the South—a new form of governance that takes seriously the emancipating potential of the struggles of health workers and researchers throughout the world.

Wellness, Modes of Living, and Styles of Living

When defining wellness, conventional mainstream social sciences and philosophy resort to an empirical approach constructed through criteria designed to analyze so-called human development and quality of life. As a result, an interminable succession of empirical constructs have been developed to describe/predict a state of personal wellness as a set of decontextualized abstractions, stripped of their historical social–cultural relations.

The New Economics Foundation(NEF) has published a review titled *Well-Being Evidence for Policy* "(Stoll, Michaelson, & Seaford, 2012). After presenting a summary of the "current literature on well-being and its determinants" structured by policy areas, NEF refer to what it considers the relative effects of different factors[13] that influence personal well-being. The account recognizes that the literature sometimes suffers from a lack of clarity regarding the use of the term *well-being*, which is used interchangeably with personal subjective well-being, life satisfaction, and happiness. Taking sides with a Cartesian individualistic–subjective perspective, it assumes that the problem is basically one of personal satisfaction (i.e., individual psychological) that varies according to determinants (i.e., factors and causes). Here, we do not return to our methodological critique of this sort of fragmented, lineal one-plane reasoning; the example here simply illustrates how this approach, notwithstanding its formal sophistication, reduces the

---

13. The proclaimed model involves an array of factors that include the economy (11 variables), social relationships and community (9 variables), health (5 variables), education and care (2 variables), the local environment (9 variables), and personal characteristics (6 variables).

complexity of wellness to a constellation of fragments organized around individual well-being and focalized governance policy.

However, as is the case with health, wellness cannot be reduced to an individual phenomena, nor can it be reduced to personal psychosocial well-being associated with empirical fragments of a personal life history. It involves a complex set of interrelated processes of society, occurring in all three dimensions of its social reproduction (i.e., G/P/I). Wellness encompasses both basic indispensable material resources and the cultural spiritual conditions—tied to the aforementioned material conditions—needed to produce a collective and individual, sustainable and supportive, psychological and spiritual sense of well-being. Epidemiology as a sociobiological science therefore requires the understanding of complex systems. It needs to incorporate complex thinking in order to explain the actual material relations and contradictions between healthy, supportive, and protective processes, which are affected or contradicted by unhealthy, hazardous processes, in all three dimensions.

Viewing this challenge from the standpoint of critical epidemiology implies embedding the notion of wellness in a substantially different conceptual and social foundation. Most important, it needs to be inscribed in a whole new life philosophy and ethos. Restating wellness is consequently a road to reshaping the struggle for new, healthy, equitable modes of living and redefining the criteria for evaluating the advancement of collective health.

To transcend the predominant individual psychological connotation of wellness from a holistic epidemiological perspective, we need to go beyond individual well-being related to empirically defined satisfaction. Wellness in fact denotes the cultural–spiritual embodiment of a material healthy social reproduction. In this sense, it is an important component of health in the paradigm of critical epidemiology. Wellness therefore entails both a material embodiment of protective, supportive, empowering, safe, satisfactory, healthy modes and styles of living—that successfully overcome the contradictory elements of destructive, undermining, alienating, and unhealthy ones—and a subjective cultural and spiritual proactive embodiment that springs from satisfaction related to safe, rewarding, pleasurable, creative, collective and personal activities. From this perspective, wellness is the collective or personal expression of fruitful social reproduction that is embodied in interrelated forms. Objective processes related to what we have called the four S's of wellness/living—sustainability, sovereignty, solidarity, and security (integral biosecurity)—constitute an indispensable foundation (Table 2.3). Accordingly, beyond material wellness, it entails coherent forms of cultural–spiritual dimensions of human existence. Among other things, this involves a profound and respectful relationship with Nature and collective equitable relations with others.

The sociohistorical development of wellness is a continuing process that is built, rebuilt, and perceived in social spaces where work, leisure, consumption, collective organization, and cultural emancipation take place in health-promoting territories. Societies of authentic wellness fight to sustain and multiply from an intercultural perspective the crucial components of living well through safe, rewarding, pleasurable, and creative collective and personal activities.

Having characterized our civilization as the antithesis of collective wellness, the horizon could be perceived as gloomy. Nonetheless, the growing awareness and global upheaval of the peoples do give rise to cautious optimism.

Table 2.3 **Principles of Good Living and Requisites for Wellness—the Four S's of Life**

Dimensions	Description
Sustainability	Capacity for present and future reproduction of human and natural life (i.e., social subject and nature)
Sovereignty	Autonomy in the conduct of a chosen social system and way of life Control of present indispensible resources and planning
Solidarity/ organicity	Equitable civilization Protective logic for the common good Organic popular organization around auto determined strategic interests Validity and feasibility of rights Solidary, psychological fraternity, and spiritual sense of well-being and togetherness Profound and respectful relation with Nature and collective equitable relations with the others
Security of life (human—ecosystem)	Healthy spaces and processes Protectors Healthy forms of embodiment

Latin American societies with a strong presence of indigenous cultures do provide some motives for optimism. A critical, academic, emancipatory paradigm related to society, life, and health can easily be harmonized with the philosophy and the principles of indigenous peoples' knowledge, their harmonious ecosensitive ways of relating to Mother Nature, and their community-based ethos that replaces competitiveness with sharing and mutual provision. This complementarity that I proposed in a previous essay (Breilh, 2003a) was effectively verified in meetings with native peoples' organizations held at Simon Bolívar Andean University (2007). In effect, during the preparatory intercultural process prior to the Constituent Assembly that would formulate a project for a new Ecuadorian constitution, the role of integral wellness (i.e., *buen vivir* or *Sumak Kawsay* in the indigenous Kichwa language) and the rights of nature were inscribed as key elements of the right to health. Consequently, there is a powerful, straightforward coherence between the assumed philosophical preeminence of human and cultural rights over business; the integral, heuristic, taxonomic, and ecosophical principles of the indigenous vision; and the conceptual ethical framework of critical epidemiology.

The dialectic of collective and individual life in concrete, social, and territorial spaces is fundamental to our critical approach. Different societal groups operate according to specifically structured living patterns for their social reproduction. In those configurations, there is a permanent opposition between healthy and unhealthy trends. So the broader social relations of society determine the life of groups, and these determine the individual styles of living[14] of their members (Table 2.4). These specific particular modes of living concur either with typical patterns of exposure and

---

14. The expression "styles of living" applied here to individual everyday itineraries is used with the intention of differentiating it from the commonly used notion of lifestyles, which in common English suggests a collective cultural trait.

Table 2.4 Collective Modes of Living and Individual Styles of Living

Characteristics	Modes of Living (Collective)	Styles of Living (Individual)
GENERAL		
Living patterns determined by class–gender–ethnic relations, structured conditions and spaces, and variations with time	Collective socially determined specific patterns of the group	Individual socially determined specific patterns of the person
Work	Space and typical conditions of the class at work: position in the productive structure; protective (healthy) and destructive (unhealthy) work patterns; exposure and vulnerability patterns	Personal labor itinerary, labor relations and protective and unhealthy socio-environmental conditions during the workday and its leisure periods
Consumption	Spaces and typical consumption patterns conditions of the class: quality and access to consumer goods; type of income; constructions of necessity; access system to goods; protective and unhealthy patterns of consumption; food and consumer goods biosecurity	Personal protective and unhealthy patterns of consumption: in food; rest and leisure periods; home place; access and quality of vital goods, services and recreation–leisure

Table 2.4 Continued

Characteristics	Modes of Living (Collective)	Styles of Living (Individual)
Organization and supports	Organizational spaces and conditions; collective, community, and family life supports and protections; political spaces and means (degrees of empowerment and resources in terms of public–social leadership, social control, and public and private accountability over class interests); union and objective capacity for the class and its empowerment	Personal capacity to organize actions in defense of health of the individual, immediate family, and at work; affective and material personal supports; formal or informal membership of class and community organizations
Cultural–spiritual means	Spaces for building sovereign culture and subjectivity; objective ability of the group to create and reproduce cultural values and identity (class, gender, and ethnicity "for themselves") linked to their strategic interests; critical thinking and intercultural development; emancipated and emancipating forms of spirituality	Individual subjectivity profile and personal identity; personal conceptions and values; critical capacity and spirituality
Metabolic relations	Society-Nature metabolism spaces; quality, sustainability, and security of the group's ecological relationships	Personal metabolic itinerary and quality of individual ecological settings.

vulnerability to harmful conditions or with characteristic capabilities for taking advantage of favorable processes and building protective immunity. In those specific contexts, individuals develop their possible personal–familiar styles of living that are finally embodied in corresponding phenotypic, genotypic, and psychological characteristics (Breilh, 1977, 2003a).

Bourdieu's (1998, p. 61) notion of *habitus*, which implies a "modus operandi," a conceptual stand that orients and organizes practical life, is only partially approximate to our understanding of modes of living. Our idea of modes of living not only encompasses an enduring cultural disposition that characterizes and contributes to molding the living patterns of a specific group but also fundamentally involves the material socio-economic basis of such cultural determination. The typical working and consumption patterns of the working class, for instance, not only depend on and develop according to their cultural and moral mold but also, among other things, are strongly determined by the material structure, timing, impositions, salary, and concrete material options of the working-class journey.

However, it is evident that the notion of the social determination of health that I described extensively for the first time in 1977 (Breilh, 1977, 1979) is the backbone of critical epidemiology. It subsequently appeared in several works by other authors belonging to Latin American social medicine and collective health movements. Together with the other categories that constitute a potent conceptual arsenal, since our work began in the 1970s, the social determination of health paradigm has been instrumental in promoting a theoretical, methodological, and practical break with the empirical–functionalist public health paradigm (Figure 2.6).

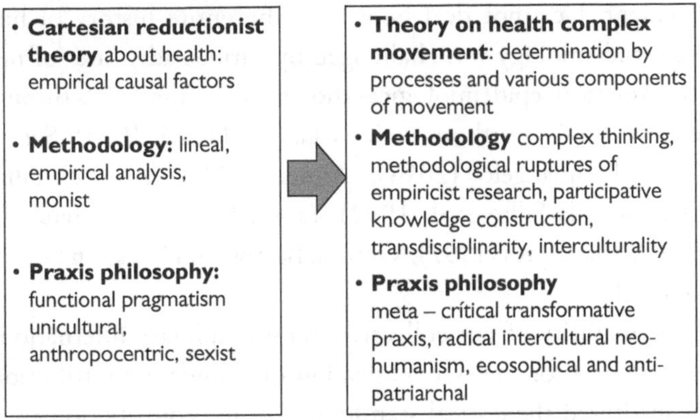

- **Cartesian reductionist theory** about health: empirical causal factors

- **Methodology:** lineal, empirical analysis, monist

- **Praxis philosophy:** functional pragmatism unicultural, anthropocentric, sexist

- **Theory on health complex movement**: determination by processes and various components of movement

- **Methodology** complex thinking, methodological ruptures of empiricist research, participative knowledge construction, transdisciplinarity, interculturality

- **Praxis philosophy** meta – crítical transformative praxis, radical intercultural neo-humanism, ecosophical and anti-patriarchal

Figure 2.6 Comparative elements of paradigm shift.

In the next section, we profile the fundamental logic and conceptual transformations that must be implemented.

Subsumption of Processes Instead of Conjunction of Factors

As discussed previously, in order to develop a new methodology, critical realism had to break with quantitative and qualitative reductionist empiricism. Five decades ago, in their critical reflections on modern teleological reason, the radical thinkers of the prolific Frankfurt School confronted its profound interpretative flaws. Habermas (1973) stated that "the social sciences that operate through the empirical analytical methods, define social reality as a system constituted by a functional connection of empirical regularities" (p. 222).

This breakup entailed a split with the interrelated static notions of causality and single-plane linearity through the conception of determination and complexity as the conditions of permanent movement. I do not deal here with the entire history of how linear epidemiology was challenged by various advocates of new Latin American epidemiological thought from the 1970s through the early 2000s—authors such as Laurell (1976, 1994), Samaja (1997), Donnangelo (2014), Almeida-Filho (Almeida-Filho, 2000; Almeida-Filho et al., 1992), Tambellini (1978), Menéndez (1998, 2008), Ayres (1997), Victora, Barros, and Vaughan (1992), and myself.

The maturity of our collective transdisciplinary international work allowed for the systematization of abundant contributions that instituted the critical standpoint. In my contribution to an international seminar in 2014, I announced a panoramic view of what I considered representative epidemiological paradigms (Breilh, 2015). Applying an analytic matrix, I classified the emblematic contributions that have influenced the development of critical Latin American epidemiology according to their ontological assumptions, epistemological transformative elements, and proposed practical (praxis) transformations. The idea was to understand the transformative performance of each school in conceptual, methodological, and ethical terms and their proximities or distances with respect to the causal empiricist schools. Here, we provide the reader with our final classification, which illustrates the diverse and enriching contributions originating in different social cultural and geographical settings (Figure 2.7).

Speaking about our contributions from the South to the refounding of contemporary critical epidemiology, we can say that they sprang from the academic and political process of the conflictive and demanding years from the late 1970s to the present. The broader outline of this progression has been widely documented and

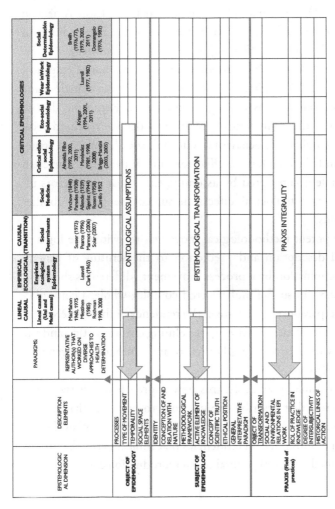

Figure 2.7 Matrix for epistemological comparative analysis of epidemiological paradigms.

Breilh, J. (2013). *Proyecto de investigacion sobre la teoria de la determinacion social de la salud la critica de la nocion del "buen vivir."* Quito, Ecuador: Fondo de Investigacion de la Universidad Andina Simon Bolivar.

commented on (Duarte Nunes, 1986; Franco et al., 1991; Waitzkin et al., 2001), and I have also summarized it in "Latin American Critical Epidemiology," which forms part of the latest edition of *Epidemiology: Political Economy and Health* (Breilh, 2010).

Being the organizing temporal–spatial metaphor of empirical epidemiological inquiry, linearity implies accepting a single-plane order of conjunctions among phenomenon. Regarding disease generation, the conjunction[15] of various decontextualized "risk factors" (individual, behavioral, cultural, social, and even structural) and their biological effect on individuals. The Cartesian logic circle is completed by assuming that those risk factors ultimately have biological effects in susceptible peoples' bodies and minds.

One potent methodological move was to switch the logic of factorial description and prediction to the scrutiny of generative determination by a process movement (differences shown in Figure 2.5). In such a multifaceted complex whole, a contradictory interplay develops between the tendency of the whole system to reproduce itself, conserving its defining characteristics, and the tendency of its parts to apply their relative autonomy to generate changes (Samaja, 1996).

As explained previously, this new approach entails switching from factors that describe conjunctions to processes that explain movement. The dialectic thrust of this movement implies the opposition of subsumption tendencies that subject particular groups to the broader logic of general social reproduction conditions, and

---

15. *Conjunction* refers to external causal links; it is fully discussed later.

singular individual living styles to the broader logic of their classes' mode of living. But, at the same time, the contrary relative auto-nomic movement of individuals in relation to their groups and of groups in relation to their society as a whole is the essential trait of the permanent transformation of epidemiological conditions.

In defining how to avoid that empiricist ontology and its epis-temological failure of not introducing the logic of determination, one central methodological problem is how to replace linear ex-ternal conjunction of factors with the inherent determination process by subsumption. As previously argued, subsumption[16] entails the conditioning of a less complex movement by a more complex one. This is not a unidirectional mechanical relation-ship but, rather, a dialectic movement that is counteracted due to the relative autonomy and generative potentiality of less com-plex processes. But subsumption generates concrete forms or embodiments that form part of the process and exhibit concrete dynamic relations between them, as demonstrated in Chapter 3 with an illustrative case. We have included the idea of embodiment (i.e., metaphorical incarnation) to complete our epidemiological reasoning. Krieger proposed to explain how we "incorporate, bio-logically, in societal and ecological context, the material and social world in which we live" (Krieger, 2011, p. 214). We realized that it was undoubtedly an important interpretative tool to explain

---

16. *Subsumption* is a general principle of existence that involves the conditioning of a less complex movement by a more complex one. It must be differentiated from the particular social historical Gramscian notion of *hegemony* that entails a form of social oppression and control of a dominant ruling sector that results from the system's seduction of subor-dinate social classes that accept and adhere to the system's logic.

the social–biological determinant relation that we presupposed in our explanation of subsumption (Breilh, 1977). The notion of embodiment completed our reasoning, but we also realized that, in our opinion, it could be extrapolated to other sorts of "incarnations" (metaphorically speaking)—that is, concrete perceptible formal expressions of those processes that go beyond the individual human body and mind. These other forms derive from critical processes that are generated at different moments of the social determination of health movement, and they are not exclusively of a personal biologic corporal or psychological nature. So we are in no way discarding Krieger's valuable contribution; on the contrary, we are applying its potent significance to other forms that necessarily participate when we assume the multidimensional complexity of the social determination process. This is because from our perspective, the notion of embodiment not only applies to the individuals "embodied in flesh." Embodiment can also represent the concrete "incarnations" that can appear as typical collective human patterns; in natural and artificialized ecosystems; or in the form of institutional, cultural, and political stable dispositions that accompany the specific social movement being analyzed. So embodiments are also generated in the particular and general domains. To explain the crucial methodological implications of this finding, S includes a graphic representation.

Chapter 3 provides an illustrative case example related to the critical processes involved and the methodological breaks we have developed in the study of the social determination of vector-borne dengue in an agro-industrial territory. Then, accordingly, it explains the practical model shifts simplified for concrete effective action.

3 | NEW METHOD AND INTERCULTURAL AWAKENING

BEYOND THE "KNOWLEDGE ILLUSION" OF THE CARTESIAN BUBBLE

Illustrative Research: Critical Processes and Methodological Break—The Social Determination of Vector-Borne Dengue in an Agro-Industrial Territory

Endemic vector-borne dengue (CIE-10 A90) is an endemic transmissible disease problem in Latin America. Its expansion in an agro-industrial territory can help us illustrate the interpretative and practical contrast between empiricist lineal and critical epidemiology. In the limited space of this section, we discuss some main differences in order to highlight the alternative methodology our research adopted.[1]

Taking advantage of our previous research experience, our university proposed to our University of British Columbia partners a study for "meeting capacity-building and scaling-up challenges

---

1. Matrix review co-authors: Luiz Allan Kunzle; María José Breilh; María de Lourdes Larrea; Bayron Torres; Doris Guilcamaigua; and Giannina Zamo.

to sustainably prevent and control dengue in the Southern Pacific coastal tropical forest of Ecuador (Machala), Ecuador—the world's main banana for export region." The idea was a join effort to investigate the effectiveness and feasibility of applying and scaling up an alternative approach to the prevention and control of dengue, which was experiencing a resurgence in this vulnerable setting. It was a successful cooperation, conducted in collaboration with Dr. Jerry Spiegel, the Canadian co-director of the project.

Based on that experience and further developments with regard to our research, I chose this case of alternative dengue epidemiology in order to illustrate the importance of the methodological breaks we have proposed. With that in mind, I recently brought together members of the interdisciplinary team of our Collective Health Impacts Research Center—Health Sciences Area of Universidad Andina Simón Bolívar of Ecuador(UASB-E), a valuable group of young researchers and doctoral students—in order to submit for discussion a perfected version of my critical process matrix as a scientific framework for an integral health impacts evaluation model (Breilh, 2019).

The exercise acknowledged the importance of the empirical elements involved as valuable knowledge tools, but it reinserted them in the complex multidimensional movement that critical epidemiology provides, to recover their epistemic potentiality.

Typically, conventional experts would condense the important epidemiological experience in communicable vector-borne diseases in a causal model to correlate "risk factors" and "outcome morbidity." We had to deconstruct such empirical lineal assortment, which frequently takes the form of a causal model reflected in a simple linear regression system. For instance, one that links independent causal variables (risk factors: x_1 = parasite; x_2 = vector; x_3 = exposure habits; x_4 = susceptibility/vulnerability; x_5 = health system resources; x_6 = community and personal supports; x_7 = environmental factors) can describe and predict the frequency and probability of the dependent variable (y = dengue indexes).

Classically, to focus the complexity of the phenomenon, but maintain the same paradigm and conjunction logic, one could develop a more elaborate design applying a multilayer, multivariate, or factorial model. Doing so would augment the formal mathematical complexity, but it would not supersede the limitations and distortions of empiricist analysis, which we have already described. At any level of formal complexity, the essential problem of linearity and functional thinking would remain.

Recent epidemic transmission models have used complex mathematical modeling tools, compartmental or stochastic, such as non-autonomous ordinary differential equations or multivariate spatial linear regression models, generating models whose resolution can only be performed using complex computational numerical methods. The results, even with high mathematical precision, are inaccurate because they are not able to take into account currently fundamental determining processes. Despite the fact that researchers often recognize these limitations, recent surveys (Brauer, 2017) indicate that future research will continue to use this conception of complexity, applying a greater number of variables and risk factors. But contrarily, our opinion is that it would be much more useful, in terms of explanatory knowledge and public policies, if the search for complexity were directed to create models that relate critical processes and the dimensions of social determination.

It is important to consider here that when we criticize empiricist causal factor logic, we are not implying that causal relations and factor incidence do not exist. What we mean is that these factors are not the exclusive nor the decisive elements of health determination; their causal incidence is defined, limited, and moderated by the conditioning force of collective modes of living and general processes.

That is because the reduction of any health problem to linear single-plane unidimensional or multidimensional relations of quantitative indicators (or nonquantitative elements derived from qualitative research) constitutes the central fetishism of the empirical epidemiological method. This logic supposedly provides an objective, calculable, and precise reflex of the true characteristics of health as an empirical construct, but its fetishist scheme disguises the social relations of those empirical facts (rates—indicators or qualitative segments) and their formal correlations.

According to its advocates, the methodological consistency of empirical analysis supposedly resides in its capacity to obtain a reliable empirical register (i.e., direct reflection of perceived phenomena) and to extract from it a valid inference—one considered to be equivalent to a scientific truth about the essence of the observed reality. The accuracy of this logic is supposed to be guaranteed by the correspondence principle (i.e., reliable registration and valid inference). According to this line of reasoning, the maximum validity criterion is the experiment or quasi-experiment, as it would be assumed as a supposedly faithful reflex of perceived reality and the most persuasive way to demonstrate the functional connection of factual regularities. Mathematical analysis is the fundamental instrument for that interpretive construction. For the sake of coherence, in order to complete that argumentative cycle, mathematical functional connections must be established that corroborate factual conjunctions through tests of association, correlation, concomitant variation, analysis of variance, factor analysis, and others. Let us look at the implications of this argument in our illustrative case.

Returning to the specificities of endemic dengue, an interesting review of conventional literature on infectious disease transmission properly recognizes some unique preconditions of the parasite and of the individual host: *transmission* from one host to another and *infectiousness* as a characteristic of a host that can infect another human (Holloran, 1998). According to Holloran, in the case of dengue, transmission entails an *infective source* determined by parasite traits (i.e., those of any of four types of arbovirus: DEN1–DEN4) such as virulence or speed with which it affects an infected human host, its replication speed in the female mosquito's organism, and the reproduction capacity of the vector insect (i.e., *Aedes aegypti*). *Exposure* is the second empirical element of transmission and is defined by contact patterns (i.e., the form of the relationship between a potentially infective host and a susceptible one), mixing patterns of infective and susceptible hosts, and the degree and duration of infectiousness. The process of herd immunity and the corresponding transmission probability mediate exposure.

In the same line of observation, infectiousness depends on the presence of infected hosts and the conditions of *susceptibility* (resistance to infection) that defines the basic reproductive number (i.e., the expected number of new hosts that infected hosts can produce during their infective period), plus the core population or group with the highest reproductive number.

Finally, regarding the clinical individual aspect of the problem, Holloran (1998) defines a first latent period of incubation, an infectious or symptomatic period, and a non-infectious period.

Undoubtedly, these observations are important valid scientific evidence, the problem being that Cartesian thinking dilutes their powerful implications in the search for real integral understanding of transmission and infectiousness. Causal descriptions and predictions lack a generative explanation and disengage each of those elements from their determinant context. It is therefore necessary to analyze and reconnect them from the social determination perspective.

In that sense, a paradigm shift is inevitable, and for this purpose we have developed new concepts and alternative fieldwork tools. Our research team's epidemiological experience of health assessment in urban and rural communities was important in strengthening our illustrative case.

A starting point was to substitute the risk factor logic with the dialectic notion of critical processes, a methodological shift that demanded a clear definition of a *critical process*, the redefinition of *variable*, and the conception and role and the creation of an alternative analytical instrument that we called the *critical process matrix*. To replace lineal heuristics, we also had to reconceive the notion of health *inequity* in order to grasp the radical contrasts among the modes of living of different class–gender–ethnic population strata. Statistical and qualitative observation techniques had to be reinterpreted to disengage them from the empiricist linearity. The choice of variables to be observed, or qualitative elements, and the mathematical techniques to be used must be established from the critical processes and within the scope defined in the general (G), particular (P), and individual (I) dimensions.

Because our matrix needs to be territorially positioned, it was also fundamental to reframe spatial determination, breaking with the Cartesian conception of a passive formal geographical health space. Finally, our evaluation matrix is intended for collective health action, implying a shift from conventional passive state-centered health surveillance to participative community-based strategic health monitoring.

The Critical Process Matrix: An Interpretative Tool of the Movement of Social Determination

A *critical process* is a multidimensional socially determined transformation that generates concrete collective and individual health and ecosystem embodiments in a particular social space and according to class, gender, and ethnocultural distribution.

Through a complex process of subsumption, the general, particular, and individual transformations positively or negatively affect specific communities. The social, ethnic, and gender organizations, plus the public health sector, can therefore respond, either to enhance or promote the positive or counteract to prevent or repair the negative. But of course this movement of social determination and concrete embodiments needs to be explained before well-informed, fair, and intercultural preventive, precautionary, and health-promoting actions are implemented.

Expanding this argument, we can say that conflicting health-promoting and unhealthy trends compete to define the actual state of healthiness in a concrete evaluated territory. In operation, critical processes include those inscribed in the general domain (G) of a defined territory, moving and evolving along the contradictions of the particular (P) modes of living of existing collectivities and their favorable and unfavorable social and metabolic relations, which in turn finally subsume the styles of living of individuals (I) who participate in those communities through their unique daily life activities and metabolism patterns. Critical epidemiology must expose both the configuring elements of the social determination process and the key embodiments and their relations. All this complex movement is at the heart of collective health, involving lever ideas, updated scientific and technical knowledge, and social organization.

Organizing participative intercultural transdisciplinary research for the enhancement of protective healthy processes and the transformation of unhealthy ones implies the previously mentioned interdependent tasks and for such purpose presupposes a triangle of action that, as explained later, articulates a strategic project around the implied challenges, a mobilized social block of affected and concerned peoples, and a consistent critical mass of scientific–technical knowledge and resources.

I devised the critical process matrix as a tool to rethink the methodology for the evaluation, monitoring, and comparison of the healthiness of a given territory among types of production, modes of living, and related ecosystems (Breilh, 2003a, 2017a). It was the result of many years of research in the development of an alternative methodology for the critical assessment of socially determined distribution of health (Breilh, Granda, Campaña, & Betancourt, 1983). Its initial motivation and use was the appraisal of health consequences of industrial activities on the human workforce, communities, and ecosystems. Our first encounter in this area was a research project in the northern Andes of Ecuador on the impacts of cut flowers for export in agro-industry (Breilh, 2007; Breilh et al., 2005). At that time, a crucial issue was the obsolete philosophy and methodology of epidemiological *surveillance*, as we explain later in this chapter.

Correspondingly, we worked on an alternative method for stratifying populations in order to compare them epidemiologically. Growing health inequity, a central motif of this development, is examined later. Here, it is important to explain the ideas and procedures that constitute the matrix.

The application of a critical processes matrix clarifies vital issues for the planning of integral health prevention and promotion. It also reinforces the role of the *precautionary principle*[2] in dealing with any ambiguities that tend to favor corporate interests.

The matrix allows us to reinterpret the priorities of a defined territory, the strategic interests of its communities, by applying as referential criteria the 4 S's of life relevant to the human groups and ecosystems of that territory. In short, the matrix allows us to arrive at a comprehensive knowledge of health, effectively position the social participants involved, and achieve an effective impact on healthy or unhealthy processes.

---

2. The precautionary principle states that if there is a reasonable suspicion that a process could be harmful to human life and health, if there is scientific uncertainty about its harmfulness, there is an ethical duty and responsibility to take action. In that case, we must proceed by transferring the weight of the proof from the community that suffers the problem to those whose activities are causing it, using a transparent, informed, and democratic decision-making process, which includes those affected.

It is intended to guide the social and institutional mobilization and management that are required in a territory (with its social, geographical, ecological, and even cyberspace components) in order to confront the collective health challenges. It also involves special lines of action on individual processes that are affecting people at that particular historical moment.

In our quest for a methodological alternative for studying critical processes in dengue (ICD-10 A90) transmission and control, we realized that the process implies an interdependent movement of certain critical subprocesses: social determination of transmission and infectivity; historic construction of policies and public management; development of collective and public system coping capacity; and the resulting metabolic subprocess of ecosystems— regional and local—in which social life, vectors, and their predators move. In terms of our illustrative case, it was necessary to insert the analysis of these components in the movement of social reproduction in order to recover their contextual relations. At the same time, we had to harmonize this procedure with the identification of the corresponding embodiments that we expect to be generated. The logic of these articulations is shown in Figure 3.1: in the top part, the three domains of the social reproduction movement (G/P/I); and in the bottom portion, the corresponding hypothetical representation of a dialectical spiral movement of certain complex health subprocesses and embodiments, which we explain later (e.g., P1, I1, and I2).

The specifying elements of this illustrative critical process are *exposure* and *inoculation*. They guided the deciphering of determination that goes from deteriorated territorial ecosystems and extractivist expansion to subordinate class–gender–ethnic

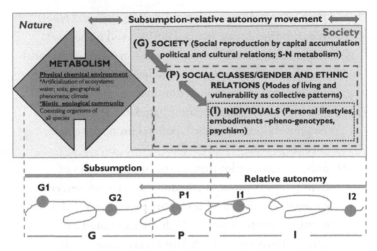

Figure 3.1 Social determination of health: articulating critical process embodiments and corresponding analytic nodes of the multidimensional critical processes in Dengue (ICD-10 A90) exposure and inoculation (Breilh, 1977, 2003a, 2015a). G, general; I, individual; P, particular.

patterns prone to dengue exposure inoculation and, finally, the high level of exposure and vulnerability to the infection and personal illness with vector-borne dengue.

The subsequent interdependent key embodiments of the critical process of dengue (ICD-10 A90) transmission are dialectically intertwined and have been depicted in five main analytic nodes:

G1: Territorial expansion of agro-industrial extractivism, chemical-based climate warming agriculture, and deteriorated metabolic conditions, generating ecosystems prone to *Aedes* reproduction; agribusiness supportive and permissive public policies and norms; chemical-based vector-borne disease control policies and norms.

G2: Expansion of small farm crisis and worsening of regional social class gap through decapitalization of small family production, imposition of dominant agricultural model, and regional segregation of urban deteriorated worker neighborhoods; municipal policies prone to vector breeding

P1: Subordinate predominant typical class modes of living (illness-prone work, domestic, consumer, educational, cultural, and transport patterns); gender and ethnic relations prone to high differentiated exposure patterns and vulnerability; class-based distribution of neighborhoods characterized by low-quality, overcrowded, socially segregated housing, limited water provision, collective patterns and conditions prone to higher dengue transmission, infective source formation, and exposure-vulnerability patterns; work ware and nutritional deficit vulnerability; limited accessibility to low-quality health care; specific metabolic relations in high-temperature, high *Aedes* density, and low predator density neighborhoods

I1: Individual styles of living and household infrastructure services provision conditions of subordinate social class members and gender–ethnic relations, which correspond to high inoculation (bite) probabilities and exposure to household breeding sites

I2: Individual human biological and psychological vulnerability and high rates of illness and dengue

> morbidity-related embodiments; entomological insect re-
> production embodiments

In methodological terms, those conglomerations constitute *analytic nodes* of subprocesses determined by historical characteristics, with their qualitative attributes of movement that are described through narratives or other elements, and quantitative characteristics or measurable traits of the examined movement and its resulting embodiments.

Because this methodology is used to understand movement and transform all determining dimensions of a critical process, our main concern is not limited to formally describing elements and predicting their measurable outcomes but, rather, to be able to explain and understand their productive or generative role in the formation of unique embodiments. Due to our critical paradigm's explanatory nature, the observational validity is not restricted to quantitative probabilistic preconditions, such as correlation or concomitant variation (i.e., a "P value").

In fact, the concept of statistical "precision" has been questioned in the scientific community because some of its parameters are also the result of arbitrary conventions, such as the P value (Ioannidis, 2018). This, in turn, calls into question the unlimited admitted use of "hypothesis contrast tests" due to random error, which, like the P value, are very dependent on the sample size (Jiménez-Paneque, 2016). The scientific community has long argued that the conclusions of a study process not only should be centered on statistical results but also should incorporate the existing knowledge on the subject under study (J. Cohen, 1994). Even in the context of the Cartesian paradigm, new approaches have been proposed, such as the use of Bayesian models in epidemiological studies. Its use, however, depends on the estimation of initial probabilities in the analysis process, based on previously accumulated knowledge.

What we propose here is to redefine the use of quantitative (statistical and other) and qualitative methods, removing variables and risk factors from the center of attention and focusing on critical processes.

Understanding the Role of Quantitative Values (Variables) and Qualitative Nodes in the Critical Paradigm

Variables in the new scheme acquire a completely different connotation. Once the integrated multidimensional subprocesses have been defined and their key embodiments emerge, we also need to extract from that movement some representative measurable variations (i.e., quantitative variables) or qualitative narrative and documental components that clearly represent or express essential dimensions of the process that can be operationalized and incorporated into the respective analytic node. This approach reframes the understanding of variables and qualitative node components in their role within the critical new paradigm. The same applies to the alternative management of all observation techniques: statistical, qualitative data, and, most important, geographic elements such as the social space of concrete territories.

The first underlying issue here is to distinguish, and at the same time relate, the *individual* and *collective* dimensions of the health process. Both count as significant sources of critical knowledge, given that dialectical reasoning does not concede epistemological primacy or exclusivity to the individual or the social totality. Although the general social reproduction system governs social movement—through the determining influence of capital accumulation—tending to reproduce the main rules of social life, individuals as well as less complex processes in the particular collective domain are nevertheless capable of relative autonomy and have the capacity to generate changes in society or in the more complex elements. In the case of collective health, the late Juan Samaja brilliantly exposed this dialectic argument. He was able to explain the complex two-way dynamism of the individual and collective health phenomenon (2005).

As I have argued in previous writings, fundamental changes must be made in the instruments and techniques of epidemiological observation to make them coherent with the new theoretical framework. Thus, for instance (Breilh, 2010),

> It becomes essential to redefine the concept of variable itself; in as much this concept is an operational bridge between the theoretical terms of the hypothesis about the processes and the tangible manifestations of the empirical phenomena involved, it is logically necessary to reformulate the dimensions and implications of the epidemiological variables. In other words, this implies rethinking the explanatory basis of the empirical foundation of scientific knowledge. (pp. 191–192)

The significance and role of epidemiological quantitative survey or qualitative interview techniques can be approached from two completely different cognitive perspectives. For the Cartesian neopositivist conception and methodology, quantitative analysis constitutes, in itself, the founding pillar of experimental or quasi-experimental quantitative correspondence observation, which at the same time is assumed as the golden rule of objectivity and the truthfulness of science. Variables, conceived of as essential measurable variations of observable particles (i.e., individual signs, symptoms or syndromes, cases, household data, etc.), are assumed to contain the essence of reality that must be reflected immaculately in a statistical or qualitative correlative empirical summary of that reality. As well from formalist qualitative perspectives such as grounded theory, empirical qualitative narrative segments constitute the pillars of phenomenological and constructivist analysis.

In other words, quantitative inductive interpretation pretends to encompass the formal regularities from which true essential knowledge would result. But looking through that interpretative optic, "true knowledge"—let alone conclusions built over reliable data registration and valid inference—is no more than a rigorous description of certain variations and their constant conjunctions, or a prediction of probable fluctuations that can be correlated with statistical software. On the qualitative side, reductionism is no more than a clustering of individual decontextualized narrative segments resulting from individual experiences that can be inductively articulated through the computer-assisted network construction of semantic relations or quantified in a semantic cloud.

Contrarily, critical methodology assumes variables or narrative segments as important expressions of an intertwined complex process. These only acquire meaning and position in relation to the social context that determines them, and the analytic node they form. In other words, the real significance and explanatory coherence of quantitative correlations or qualitative semantic segments found in empirical registers can only be established and understood in relation to the determining material conditions and cultural movement of the social space of which they form part. Conversely, they are particular dialectical quantitative or qualitative expressions of a contextual critical process movement.

The importance of considering dialectical social determination of quantifiable evidence as an ontological condition derives from two main facts. First, it entails expanding the notion of variability beyond the probabilistic form of *variance*—which corresponds to the causal conjunction movement of independent and dependent variables, their correlations and concomitant variations—to include other forms that were mentioned previously. Second, it makes possible the conversion of quantitative analysis from a rigid instrument, restricted to quasi-experimental observed correlations of empirical indicators (risk factors) and probable outcomes, to a dynamic resource that is capable of providing an objective comprehension of the explanatory power of quantitative empirical evidence. Facts related to quantity must be tied to a determinant process and are indispensible in explaining and understanding its productive or generative contribution to the shaping of the specific embodiments we are studying.

If we look back at our illustrative case on dengue, these arguments can be clarified. From a conventional standpoint, for example, assuming some entomological indexes—that is, the *A. aegypti* index, the Breteau index, and the positive breeding site index—as variables for our exercise, we could operate with them from two radically different methodologies. If the variables are reified and considered only as self-explanatory variations—respectively of the percentage of positive households, the percentage of positive breeding sites, and the percentage of positive sites in a community—one could assume them, for instance, as "risk factors" to be correlated with dengue morbidity or mortality rates. One could correlate them to "causes of the causes" to describe their presence and probability. One could also incorporate them into a multifactorial scheme to describe distribution trends. In whatever case, a scientific question—for example, How is the increasing prevalence of endemic dengue generated and socially and territorially distributed?—would be reduced by this conventional perspective to a modest or even very complex analysis of the constant conjunctions of a system of formal variables. From this perspective, one would consider their position in the network of causal ramifications and conjunctions as "independent" (i.e., "causal"), dependent, or intervening variables.

What happens in this first illustrative option is that if one assumes a variable array selected under empirical single-plane probabilistic logic, one incurs in the cycle of methodological reductionism that Bhaskar (1986) criticized, and that we previously explained, the richness and complexity of reality, which is reduced to a single plane consisting of perceivable phenomenon: the empirical pattern. Second, a pattern of conjunctions of so-called independent and dependent variables is chosen under abstract norms of significance (i.e., the golden rule of P values), putting aside nonassociative phenomena or nonsignificant conjunctions and striping out their profound dynamic connections with the generative movement. Finally, a subset of functional variables is arranged as a proxy of an experimental design and described as a closed system and considered as the representation of epidemiological reality. The empiricist cognitive sequence is then as follows: demonstrated constant conjunction = causal law = knowledge. This knowledge, as we have argued previously, is not explanatory and constitutes an extracted segment of reality that does not represent its real complexity. In other words, in collective and public health terms, it is incomplete and frequently misleading.

The use of statistics has therefore been restricted to the valuation of a decontextualized array of variables considered significant and their conjunctions arranged according to different study designs and corresponding probability tests. In empiricist epidemiological research, the golden rule is to approximate the study design to the theoretical experimental model. In the pure experiment, the researcher defines "treatment" and "control" groups and must obtain almost absolute initial group similarity in all fundamental characteristics (i.e., variables) by randomized distribution (random allocation). Then, when different "treatments" (doses) are applied in the treatment groups and placebos in the control group, one can observe conventionally defined effects and infer significant differences to demonstrate effective causality. A successful experiment is a consistent proof of a cause–effect relation and of treatment effectiveness.

For very obvious reasons, causal epidemiology cannot operate a pure experiment, but its founders have cleverly formulated three types of designs, according to the empirical analytic proximity to the experimental logic.[3] Restricting statistical design to this rationality has produced valuable findings, but at the same time has

---

3. For our argument's sake and to simplify things, the three well-known designs are (1) cross-sectional or transversal designs that are considered exploratory, (2) case–control designs (also called retrospective) that compare past exposure to hypothetical "causes" in the past of ill hospitalized cases versus non- or insignificant exposure in a hospital control population in which that illness is absent, and (3) longitudinal cohort designs that follow up initially healthy cohorts with different degrees of exposure to a suspected cause.

some undesirable implications. First, it implies adhering to the lineal reductionist conception that equates the real world with an incomplete arrangement of factual evidences and relations. Second, it adheres to the reductionist conception of the scientific method that reduces it to a logic arrangement to proof stable effective conjunctions of empirical quantitative phenomena. Third, it reduces the conception of statistics to an auxiliary technique for describing and predicting significant permanent factual quantitative connections in the framework of a probabilistic hypothesis. Seen through this reasoning, this valuable tool betrays its potential capacity to understand the contribution of quantifiable variations in the development of an epidemiological process.

Redesigning Epidemiological Statistics and Qualitative Observation

Knowledge Illusion with Precision

The "knowledge illusion" of linear reductionist thinking lies in its emphasis on building consistent formal models, detached from their contextual evaluative relations—merely describing variable associations, correlating them, and predicting their formal links and behavior under defined probabilistic conditions.

This pattern of Cartesian science placed quantification at its center. By the late 15th century, positivists positioned quantitative measurements as the central element of knowledge. In order to avoid the "noise" of social conditionings, those measurable facts had to be freed from their social connections and separated from their qualitative historical evaluative relations. This logical split was crucial for the sake of manipulating and exploiting natural processes and social relationships. It was also of great importance in transforming socially generated data into useful practical decontextualized abstractions. In logical terms, Cartesian statistics also influenced a type of social science concerned with description and prediction instead of explanation, all very convenient for the reproduction of the prospering capitalist society (Leiss, 1972). Thus, through the reductionist process of reifying and quantifying, dominant positivist science and statistics were situated as a means of pragmatic manipulation and commodification of natural and social objects (i.e., epidemiological objects), instead of a critical transformative explanation of reality.

As previously mentioned, by adopting those Cartesian principles, conventional epidemiology assumed variables as expressions of the variations that occur in individuals that move in a regular dynamic system. From there, under this conceptual and logic frame, differential equations and data assortments are assembled from individual variations and assumed as the rules of movement, and they are taken as the formal representation of reality. From this perspective, statistics mainly operates through contingencies, correlations, variance analyses, and factorial groupings of empirical "tip of the iceberg" phenomena (Breilh, 1997).

Critical reasoning consequently leads us to the conclusion that conventional applications of statistics does not study real variation but, rather, a constructed trimmed-down variation. This lineal simplification discards all types of phenomena in the social context that do not comply with strict probabilistic validity, considering them as statistical "noise." In other words, this maneuver unwillingly converts statistical operations into a reifying mechanism. But conventional lineal statistics can also create relations that do not exist by disengaging observed correlations from their context of variation; by arbitrary selection of variables; by excluding from analysis the system's history; by not considering the importance of the observation's time or considering it only in a linear, nonhistorical, way. For these and other reasons, the supposed inherent objectivity of statistical analysis by itself is inconsistent or biased, and especially in fields such as the life and social sciences, Cartesian statistics may well have become ideological embodiments (Levins & Lewontin, 1985)—a type of reductionism that substitutes reality with a formal variable scheme that passes probabilistic rules and favors functional governance.

A Crucial Challenge for Critical Methodology: Reinterpreting the Quantitative–Qualitative Dialectic

Even in some progressive academic scenarios and quite frequently in conventional public health venues, the reaction to quantitative survey empiricist monism has lent itself in many cases to a revival of cultural relativism and its new face of qualitative empiricism. Disciplines such as epidemiology, seeking an intercultural interdisciplinary approach, face a paradoxical situation: On the one hand, there is the need to consolidate an alternative epidemiological scheme that demands increasing incorporation of critical anthropological and ethnographical "qualitative methods," and on the other hand, this rapprochement has brought cultural relativism to many study designs.

Outstanding contributions have revealed the blurring consequences caused by cultural relativism and communicational ideology in the ethnographic and anthropological method components of collective health research. This is a relevant problem that Nestor García-Canclini (1993) explained when analyzing empirical anthropology and its cultural relativism. In his opinion, one serious methodological consequence is to

> analyze subaltern cultures using only the account of the authors... faithfully duplicating the informant's speech.... That naive empiricism ignores the divergence between what we think, and our practices, between the self-definition of the subaltern classes, and what we can know about their lives from the social laws in which they are inserted. (p. 71)

Also, Eduardo Menéndez, in his groundbreaking anthropological essay on alcoholism in Mexico, demonstrated that much of the contents of personal interviews simply echoed the public systems narratives (Menéndez & Di Pardo, 1996). Concomitantly, Charles Briggs and Clara Mantini have brought to our attention the cultural and logical influence of dominant ideologies and practices of communication (i.e., communicability). In their view, "Spheres of communicability in health—or biocommunicability—constitute a form of governing that creates and ranks subjectivities and social locations" (Briggs, 2005, p. 102). From their groundbreaking critical ethnographic approach, Briggs and Mantini-Briggs (2003) have revealed the complex, often neglected, class, attitudinal, and institutional relationships that are a vital component of the socio-cultural determination of health.

The critique of quantitativism and the spread of qualitative approaches, enhanced by the appearance of computer-based textual and other types of documental analysis, have stimulated the multiplication of mixed qualitative–quantitative studies (Punch, 2014; Tashakkori & Teddlie, 1998). This was a valuable move; however, the pressures of conventional phenomenological, constructivist, and pragmatist approaches have oriented it toward a dominant positivist cultural outlook.

In any case, after the prolonged rule of the empirical quantitativist paradigm in the social sciences, qualitative approaches have expeditiously developed, opening solid grounds for an integral management of empirical evidence. In the transition, a clear tension existed between qualitative and quantitative advocates, but with time, the real significance of the qualitative and quantitative inputs has contributed to a renewed organization of methodology and a sharp distinction has now been questioned (Punch, 2016). Moreover, in the Latin American critical health sciences, the critique of the quantitative–qualitative split made part of the paradigmatic shift implied in the development of collective health and critical epidemiology (Almeida-Filho, 1992; Minayo, 1992, 2009).

In order to understand the important role of quantitative and qualitative analysis in epidemiological research, but marking distance from Cartesian culturist conceptions related to the scientific method, we must re-examine some basic assumptions. Methodological design starts with the conception of the object of study, frequently named "study object." For this purpose, the indispensable categories, observational descriptors, and assumed relations are structured and developed around the object's characteristics and movement. As we have argued previously, a phenomenon that forms part of the study object needs to be understood within its context: characterizing its quantitative aspects as well as its qualitative features. That is because real processes acquire quantities in relation to given qualitative attributes. Namely, both qualitative and quantitative developments are interdependent. This being so, in order to understand the essential traits of measurable evidences, we cannot disconnect them from their qualitative historical frame. The previously mentioned methodological conclusion leads us to critically observe the shortcomings of conventional detached qualitative research. For the same reasons that we have contested the preeminence of quantitative measurement as the fundamental source in science, we must be clear that the solution to *quantitativism* is not replacing it with rationalist *qualitativism*.

The latter is a methodological principle of critical reasoning that must be extrapolated to our study designs, linking the perceived narratives with the general and particular social cultural relations. In other words, quantitative and qualitative attributes of our population and its health are not essentially individual creations but, rather, are formed and transformed under complex social determination (Breilh, 1997).

In terms of our illustrative case, the identified analytic nodes or process segments of the critical process, with their corresponding embodiments, involve articulated qualitative and quantitative expressions.

Radical Social Stratification: A New Perspective on Health Inequity

Throughout this book, we have argued that one defining characteristic of today's societies, both in the North and in the South, is a preposterous social *inequity* that brings about a profound health *inequality*—two apparently similar concepts that nonetheless entail significant differences. Inequity, in our model, refers to the mechanisms for concentration of power by a social minority and the corresponding process of exclusion of the subordinate groups with regard to the access to goods and rights. Inequality, on the other hand, is the empirical embodiment of inequity. In the case of health, the latter expresses the differences in access to elements that account for a healthy mode of living and those related to health rights and services. In other words, inequity is the essential determining characteristic of unfair distribution, and inequality is the empirical "tip of the iceberg" expression of unfairness. For instance, big business capital accumulation by the pharmaceutical and biomedical industries forms part of inequity, whereas the differential rate of access to health care services is a typical indicator of inequality.

Extreme unfairness is the characterizing societal trait of our times. In broad terms, inequity delimits the state of wellness that people can enjoy by mediating the particular quality of living modes that specific social classes are capable of experiencing. Urban and rural communities of the affluent North and of the South are radically segregated as a result of class, gender, and ethnocultural dividers that form part of class–gender–ethnic-based distribution of modes of living. The historical conditions of work and consumption patterns, empowerment and organizational protective resources, sovereign identity building, and metabolic relations with socially determined ecosystems all are typically segregated. Both the protective and harmful components of those social patterns and their contradictory movement depend on those social class–gender–ethnic relations.

In these circumstances, wellness and health are built-in global and local segregated scenarios of the concentrated opulence and technology access of minorities in certain regions and, at the same time, of ever increasing poverty, needs, and unhealthiness for the vast majority.

In the face of such a reality, Virchow's (1848) call for "radical measures and not mere palliatives" implies not only transformative science but also specific conceptual and instrumental elements that conventional epidemiology and public health do not provide. Reframing the construction of social strata is a major challenge in that regard.

In addition to the interpretative flaws related to variance, the role of variables, and the qualitative–quantitative dynamics, another fundamental failing of conventional epidemiological statistics is its social classification logic. Populations need to be constantly socially stratified for epidemiological comparison, but positivist social stratification builds strata in a way that is convenient to its rules of objectivity. This methodological reduction is obtained by separating certain categories regardless of their dialectic interdependence, to substitute the broader cognitive categories with their partial less encompassing pairs. These false-cognitive separations between ampler cognitive categories (i.e., evaluation references) and their partial descriptive expressions, which obscure sociological analysis, are inequity–inequality, production–consumption, class modes of living—individual living opportunities, and exploitation–disadvantages of opportunity.

The reduction of class-based to individual-based stratification is achieved by means of these logic separations and substitutions—first reducing and substituting the fundamental analysis of social inequity to the empirical dimension of inequality, and then replacing the analysis of determinant processes that are generated in the productive sphere and its social relations, with a descriptive account of personal consumption facts such as income and individual opportunities. The blurring of collective class relations and modes of living and their investigative replacement with individual notions, such as individual low income and the lack of opportunities, obscures the sociological assessment of unfair distribution and displaces the analytic fulcrum from the social system to the individual sphere.

We therefore need to overcome the social classification system that Cartesian logic applies. Classifications, being a "spatial or spatial–temporal segmentation of reality . . . when they become visible, [they can] become objects of contention" (Bowker & Star, 1999). In epidemiology, when we classify the population by grouping it according to empirical indicator intervals, we are applying—knowingly or not—a Cartesian social classification that completely omits essential objective social relations, certain meanings, and identities. This leads us to focus our logic on the individual dimension and to individualize health actions.

The reductionist lineal approach operates by means of social characterization survey instruments (i.e., scales) that are focused on providing an empirical social typology for epidemiological analysis.[4] With or without express intention, the obvious perceptive consequence of this type of epidemiological questionnaire is that unjust exploitive social relations are diluted and empirical results will tend to concentrate action on simply diminishing or controlling isolated empirical indicators. The overall result is that public health policies and programs are reduced to cosmetic indicator mitigation instead of fighting for sound integral transformative reform.

The INSOC Inequity-Based Social Stratification Methodology

If consistent and critical epidemiological research or planning must be based on a true interpretation of class inequity, the congruent question is: How do we study the essence of social disparity and stratify our population in order to obtain accurate social comparisons?

The "postmodern" debate about the transcendence of social class analysis in contemporary science evidences a profound clash between supporters and detractors. We are not able to deal here with the details of this important dispute. What is important for our line of epidemiological reasoning is to provide a consistent answer to the question, How do we identify and study the essence of

---

4. Unfortunately, this problem also affects the structure of the enormous databases of health services of most countries, especially of the most affected regions, because they lack social class and neat territorial information that would make them a powerful tool for alternative health planning. In this same way, private record transparency should be made compulsory. In any case, with the exception of personal identification information, public and private health care records should be made available to social control-accountancy and health planning.

social inequity that so profoundly affects wellness and collective health?

Class analysis has always been a highly contested scientific practice. Aside from some imperfections throughout its justified and diverse development, this debate reveals a polarization based on ideological and scientific pre-notions or opposition based on conservative paradigms. However, in postmodern scenarios, the urge to enhance cultural diversity, existential oneness, and the craving to challenge any narrative on collectiveness and totality as oppressive has triggered a hypercritical stand on class analysis. According to some, class analysis is "an antiquated construction of declining utility in understanding modern and postmodern inequality" (E. Wright, 2005, p. 51), denoting the negative prejudiced veil that mystifies the scientific understanding of unfair social relations. Nonetheless, the increasing visibility of social inequity in both hegemonic and subaltern societies constantly reaffirms the transcendence of instruments to assess its impacts. Putting these reflections in epidemiological terms, class analysis is clearly indispensable because it is a central element of research into the determining conditions of structured inequity. We need to understand the structural process of social segregation that systematically classifies people according to the historical quality of their modes of living, the subsequent hazardous or protective processes they systematically experience, and their resulting collective patterns of exposure and vulnerability.

In Latin America, class analysis has been subject to similar intellectual influences as those in the North, but class segregation crossed by gender and ethnic discrimination has long been a crucial issue of academic and political debate. In no way can this brief section provide a complete analysis of this fundamental matter. The objective here is to highlight the conceptual and methodological pillars of our position and the corresponding class analysis method we have been developing since 1977.

A cutting-edge book, *Approaches to Class Analysis*, edited by the late Erik Olin Wright (2005), summarizes the three broad classes of significant contributions to class analysis that complement and enrich the long-term economic–political tradition based on the social and technical relations of the production sphere.[5] Needless to say, at this point we are discarding the empirical constructs methodology because of its incongruences.

The first to be mentioned is the neo-Durkheimian tradition that contests the postmodern conservative argument that the site of production no longer generates discernible classes. From this perspective, rather than abandoning the site of production and switching to personal "attitudes and behavior" analysis, its advocates recognize the technical division of labor and the class structure of the labor market. One valuable neo-Durkheimian contribution is the need to explore microclasses (i.e., class fractions) or intermediary groups that are also meaningful.

The second, the neo-Weberian method, makes important contributions. In its conceptual center is the definition of the market as the major determinant of life possibilities. It highlights the Weberian notion that "a class situation is one in which there is a shared typical probability of procuring goods, gaining a position in life and finding inner satisfaction" (Weber, 1978, p. 302).

---

5. A tradition based on Marx's and many others' works.

According to Weber, the market and personal skills distribute those life chances. Notwithstanding Weber's important role in the development of this field of research, his emphasis on the market and personal life chances reduces the real scope of the problem. But the post-Weberian class analysis models, such as that of the Goldthorpe class schema (Erikson & Goldthorpe, 1992), do differentiate positions within labor markets and productive units by analyzing them in terms of employment relations. The Goldthorpe schema divides the population into six groups according to their contractual relations: Classes I and II consist of occupations with a service relationship of higher and lower grades of professionals and administrative and managerial workers, classes IIIa and IIIb consist of routine higher and lower grade non-manual occupations, class IV consists of the self-employed and small employers (class IVa comprises small owners with employees and class IVb comprises small owners without employees), and class V consists of lower technical and manual supervisory occupations. Undoubtedly, labor contract and service types are significant modulators of work and social living, but this classification still relies on secondary processes and does not include the primary core social relations. It is similar to the methodology that has been applied in Great Britain and its emblematic "Black Report" (Black & Whitehead, 1988; United Kingdom Department of Health and Social Security, 1982).

The third is the notable contributions of Pierre Bourdieu that eschew the reductionist approach of empirical quantitativist class analysis by amalgamating qualitative and quantitative sources. His central preoccupations were to reveal the driving force of *habitus* or dispositions that orient action (i.e., thoughts, perceptions, expressions, and conducts) and also to uncover the importance of *symbolic systems*. In his view, contrasts in social status should be interpreted as manifestations of social class differences; he also insists on the connection between class location and habitus, and habitus with consumption practices. Whatever stand we take with regard to the centrality of cultural patterns and symbolic power in his thesis, Bourdieu has provided crucial elements for the construction of critical social analysis. They are important to the social sciences, and specifically to epidemiology, because they encompass the roles of cultural and behavior dispositions in the definition of wellness while avoiding an economicist bias.

By now, this abridged synthesis may have convinced the reader about the serious failings of the empirical type of stratifications that we see in most public health mainstream journals. In one way or another, this type of analysis incurs in extreme reductionist classifications that distort socio-epidemiological research and reduce it to formal comparisons of means or proportions, secular trends, or scales built on individual indicators.

The INSOC: Social Insertion Questionnaire

As explained previously, in the late 1970s when we made public our version of a new critical complex thinking paradigm for epidemiology, we proposed two main categories as conceptual fundamentals of critical epidemiology: social reproduction (by capital accumulation) and the social determination of health. The latter involved four other fundamental cognitive elements: determination, society–nature metabolism, subsumption, and inequity (Breilh, 1977, 2010). So beginning with our initial works, we emphasized the objective imperative of examining the health impacts of unfairness and, as a consequence, the importance of collective patterns of health phenomena heavily segregated by inequitable social class relations.

In that sense, critical epidemiology considers collective health as a complex process irreducible to the health of individuals. As we have continuously argued, both collective and individual conditions intervene in the determination of health. However, although collective processes subsume individual development, they are not a simple sum of individual conditions. Precisely, class analysis makes this evident by demonstrating the existence of socially defined collectivities that have their own specificities and at the same time operate as a bridge between the social system's reproduction as a whole and the delimitation of the individual life. Social class patterns are the consequent embodiments of society's contradictions and at the same time determine the subsequent individual embodiments of its members. They allow us to discriminate between essentially different modes of living, which explain typical collective and individual health embodiments.

Social class is a vital theoretical category for understanding the modes of living of its members, defined by their typical patterns of work, family consumption, types of collective organization, forms of cultural beliefs, subjectivity, spirituality and behavior, and ecosystemic relations. Social class depends on the economic mode of insertion of its members in the dominant social reproduction apparatus of society, but it entails complex cultural, political, and even environmental relations.

What separates or congregates people in groups (i.e., social classes) and defines their degree of empowerment is the magnitude and power they possess to maintain, defend, and promote their strategic historical needs and objectives. In an approximate synthesis, social power comprises five interdependent dimensions: *economic power* (the capacity to control property and vital goods and resources and orient their use), *political power* (the capacity to convoke and mobilize the people toward defined goals, policies, and forms of public agency), *cultural–epistemological power* (autonomy and the capacity to mold identity, convenient forms of subjectivity, and symbolic forms and to empower them), *administrative power* (the capacity to define, manage, and have access to strategic resources), and *scientific power* (autonomy and the capacity to position and expand the rules of objectivity, interpretative and descriptive methods, as well as social perspectives of science linked to sovereign strategic needs).

The class structure of 21st-century societies is complex and is subject to permanent change. Because social typology is initially defined by economic insertion, due to the need to segregate distinct social characteristics for fieldwork research, we have operationalized the modes of insertion by means of a simple questionnaire termed *INSOC* (from the Spanish "inserción social").

The starting point was to assume a straightforward definition of *social insertion*: the concrete relations that demarcate people's class situation in the productive sphere. This theoretical presupposition arose from the need to overcome the logic of life chances as dependent on consumption capacity. It is evident that members of a same social class have similar consumption patterns and chances, but their drastic social segregation arises primarily from their economic insertion and the corresponding type of quota of collective wealth that their insertion entitles them to enjoy.

Classical political economy establishes the relations that characterize and separate social classes: (1) place in the productive apparatus through an occupation's position; (2) technical relationship with means of production defined by role in the organization of work; (3) property relations in reference to means of production; and (4) distribution relationships, defined by the share or quota of collective wealth that the specific insertion entitles them to enjoy (Illich, 1966).

Armed with that definition, our next step was to operationalize the category's relations for (1) direct field survey work or (2) secondary data classification (reprocessing). We do not further expand our explanation here; rather, we refer readers to some basic bibliography.

For the first application, our bibliography describes the structure of the corresponding social insertion module of digital or physical epidemiological survey questionnaires; explains the survey items (i.e., simple, straightforward questions related to each of the relations mentioned previously and the corresponding coded answer scales); and displays the algorithms for computer-based classification and the validation of questionnaires (Breilh, 1989, 2017b). It also provides some chosen publications of research in local communities (Breilh, 1993a, 2018b; Breilh, Pagliccia, & Yassi, 2012) or large-scale national surveys (Ministerio de Salud y Protección Social de Colombia, 2014). Also, the INSOC model has been useful for extracting a social class composition from census data at different territorial scales: local, parish, county, province, and national. It applies a social class classification algorithm using census items that the international censal forms employ, which constitute a proxy of the four classificatory categories or social relations that we explained previously: status or productive position, technical control of productive means, property of means, and income source. To test the method's accuracy, we have compared the classification it yields with that obtained in the same territory by the INSOC survey. In Colombia, an advance version of the model has been successfully applied to classify the population of national databases that use censal coding (Otálvaro, 2019).

Reframing Spatial Determination: Breaking with the Cartesian Conception of the Health Space ("Medical Geography")

One of epidemiology's basic tools is health geography, conventionally designated by the more limited label of medical geography.

Whether for practical productive purposes or for ideological reasons, knowledge is basic to the construction of socially defined ways of living and the advancement of policies. The potency of this feature has led to scientific work being submitted to the permanent pressure of economic and political power. Epidemiology, with its taxonomies, relationships, comparisons, and measurements related to social and workforce conditions and the associated environment, is an appetizing tool. Geography, with its maps, empirical geographic systems, and graphic corematic elements, also allows for sociospatial patterns to be determined. Nonetheless, these constructions depend on the applied theoretical paradigm (Ziman, 2002).

Scientific development is therefore continuously subject to epistemological scrutiny and conceptual skirmish. Geographical science in particular has been the subject of an epistemological debate between those who sponsor and work from a sociohistorical space perspective and advocates of the Cartesian conception of space. Under the latter umbrella, its role in epidemiological studies is conceived as merely describing an external "place" (i.e., map) where physical, social, and environmental health "factors" and population can be located. In classic and contemporary modern digital empiricist cartography, this approach reduces space to a passive container where natural, economic, cultural, or social phenomena are displayed in one plane or in multiple layers. The geographical landscape is taken as a passive container of natural accidents, animals, and forms of vegetation or human-made constructions.

The Cartesian perspective of science surfaced in 18th-century Europe. The convergent material demands of the industrial revolution and its need for a new social ethos and modes of living came together with the expansion of the Protestant daily life ethic in preparing societies for the new social discipline. At that time, scientific thinking was the exception and had to be adapted to the logic of a nascent industrialism and its new civilization. Correspondingly, academic institutions began to forge suitable ideas of space, time, distance, and health, destined to reaffirm the new capitalist order and its demands of descriptive knowledge of resources, places, distances, and other types of measurable means. This implied a class of science that assumed as truthful and rational whatever results that suited the dominant notion of objective spatial "normality" and "progress" (Breilh, 2010).

Within the framework of the construction of colonial power, geography was important in developing commercial routes and defining strategic spaces and even in tracing the cartography of conquest. Geographical categories were applied to the organization of colonial territory. The center–periphery relationship made possible the establishment of a hierarchic cartography. The line was necessary to demarcate property and the conquered territories. The notion of center positioned governance power within the territorial system, whereas periphery located the subaltern territories as remote and outside the aforementioned center (Smith, 1999). When the geographical globe was unfolded into a single-plane *mappae mundi,* an arbitrary North appeared and the land extensions of hegemonic countries of the North were augmented. This sort of spatial bias has been inscribed into the current sophisticated systems of geographical analysis.

As Lefebvre (1991) has explained, space came to be understood as nothing more than a "passive locus" of social relations instead of an active process that participates in their determination. Cartesian analysis has concealed these social relations and also the fact that the social space of reproduction reinforces and determines them in many ways.

Broadly speaking, Cartesian geography conveniently constructs and makes visible in various layers certain places, locations, distances, pathways of mobility, and spatial organization. Geographical constructs are no more than spatial relations of designated empirical objects. Geography is merely a spatial classification tool. Space is solely a mental metaphor for empirical situations. As explained previously, Cartesian logic is characterized by systematic and distorting separations or dichotomies, one very important separation being that of geography and history, which creates a false divide between geographic space and its historical context (M. Santos, 1985, 1996).

Thus, social space participates as a material condition of human and natural forms of life. It is very important to realize that the historical development of inequity "is not only constructed and reproduced through inequitable production and market relations, but correspondingly through the determining influence of a material organization of life, of a social model that organizes the practices of living" (Breilh, 2011, p. 390). In other words, the intermediating role of spatial determination is fundamental.

David Harvey (2007) explains that Cartesian geography, by fragmenting and reifying reality, also fragments geographical knowledge. Paraphrasing Harvey, we can therefore affirm that in order to account for the complexity and concatenation of collective health processes, our conception of geographical space must supersede the aforementioned empiricist notion. Critical geography of health must become holistic and assume dialectical thinking related to the contradiction between healthy and unhealthy spatiality.

As we have previously asserted, descriptive empirical geography considers geographical locations (i.e., places) as the "passive locus" of health factors, in one or several layers, instead of explaining them as historical embodiments that articulate certain material and symbolic configurations (i.e., forms of localization, the urban or rural distribution of phenomena). The reductionist logic of empirical geography generates descriptive cartographies heavily influenced by dominant interests. Consequently, the empirical geography of health limits itself to describing the spatial distribution of risk factors or health indicators, stripping place and factors of their historicity, movement, and contradictions. Concomitantly, Cartesian health geography simply distributes people or populations according to certain attributes and then correlates them to the said risks or causes empirically present in those particular places. Complex, multidimensional, and contradictory processes are ignored and geographical relationships are drained of their significance as health-determining processes. As previously mentioned, the Brazilian geographer M. Santos (1985) acutely explained this conceptual masquerading as a separation of history and geography.

The underlying theoretical basis of critical geography can be found in Lefebvre (1991, 2007), Harvey (2007), and M. Santos (1996). For epidemiology, incorporating their potent contributions is crucial to understanding the relationship between space, time, life, productive and living modes, and subsequently health, from a different perspective.

Geography clearly participates in the determination of social phenomena and social relations. Geographical space is not merely the medium for social activities and relations, nor a "mere aggregate of the procedures used in their dismantling." Through a historical process, social space has evolved into many forms. Each form presents its own properties, connections, networks, relationships, and dynamics. Social spaces interpenetrate and superimpose each other—a notion that supersedes the abstract view of classical mathematics (Euclidean/Cartesian) (Lefebvre, 2007). Later, we argue that the main forms of social space are geographical, ecosystemic, and, more recently, cybernetic.

Epidemiology and geography coincide because our modes of living are inscribed in space–time relations and in turn contribute to the determination of society's time and spatial configurations. Not only the material forms of space and time but also the ideological and symbolic–cultural configurations determine our modes of living (Herrera, González, & Saracho, 2017). In other words, the social determination of health has a territorial basis. This dialectic relation is related to the historical construction of the healthiness or unhealthiness of the spaces of social reproduction

Social reproduction in our societies operates on the basis of inequitable wealth accumulation and therefore requires the pre-eminence of dominant relations and hegemony. People must act and think accordingly in order to organize production and the circulation of merchandise (i.e., a consumer society). But that movement also demands compatible forms of spatiality needed to support, or prop up (as it would be called in Lefebvrian terms), the system. These spatial configurations and dynamics are profoundly related to social structures and our modes of living and our collective health (Figure 3.2). The system's reproduction entails not just things that make it function and sustain and support it. It needs a functional culture that induces collective acceptance and agreement. But none of the previous elements would suffice if it were not for an adequate functional spatial configuration. The system requires forms, functions, locational structure, mobility, and communication that maximize the feverish search for exponential increases in profit rates.

All this being said, we come to understand that life and space are accordingly imprisoned by the logic of the vicious cumulative cycle that fuels our societies. Places and services are valued and qualified according to postal codes that correspond to different social classes. Their connectivity and mobility are configured

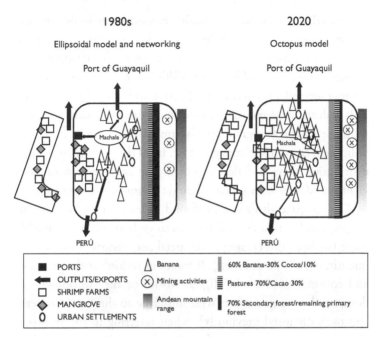

Figure 3.2 Historical redistribution of sociospatial patterns: corematic map of extractivist and unhealthy metabolism expansion (Based on: G. Zamora. 2020. Doctoral dissertation, Andina University).

accordingly. Transformations of urban and rural landscapes respond to hierarchies and priorities modeled to serve the strategic interests of big business. The process of spatial segregation generates symbolic elements that are promoted or discarded according to their favorable or unfavorable implications for the interests of the dominant groups in a determined territory (Herrera et al., 2017). Expanding spatial inequity is permanently challenging critical geography to become, as now, the geography of inequity.

The critical geography of health consequently builds its perspective based on complex thinking and assumes space as an active element of the dialectical organization of society's reproduction; it constitutes the material location of life in movement and the permanent interrelation between collective and individual processes. This dialectic movement is socially determined as much as a determining element. Geographical dynamicity also entails the metabolic scenarios our societies generate. In all this movement, spatial distribution plays a dialectic role in the construction of both healthy and unhealthy social–natural territories and landscapes.

Digital space also has a profound impact on life, and in our geographical analyses this obliges us to go beyond "real," tangible space (without this ceasing to be social and historical and, consequently, socially determined). It forces us to look at the processes and contradictions of the digital world, or the "world-net" (as designated by some authors who subscribe to the "world system" approach discussed previously), when referring to the atomized virtual territory of connected nodes. Geography must therefore go beyond conventional maps and cartographies.

Cyberspace Determination: The Fifth Subsumption of Life

In recent decades, new forms of the determination and conditioning of life have emerged in the cybernetic domain. The social relations of our "direct" world that have always challenged the critical sciences are now being multiplied in cyberspace. No matter from which theoretical–epistemological or ideological–political horizon we approach this issue, there is growing evidence of corporate dominance in cyberspace. The new digital technological revolution that big business governs allows corporations to expand the profitable cyber extractivism of collective and individual daily life. Some frightening facts are appearing that imply the advent of an era of radical, unhealthy subsumption of life processes in the virtual pole of our 21st-century modes of living.

In our contribution to the IX Brazilian Epidemiology Congress, we proposed incorporating the cybernetic dimension of the social determination of health (Breilh, 2015). This is not the place to examine this matter in detail but, rather, to emphasize the relevant emergence of a new dimension of the social determination of health, one that opens up the fifth subsumption of life. Figure 3.3 is a conceptual map that articulates the key concepts of social spatiality.

We have already spoken about the conceptualization of social space and its different forms or subdimensions. Moreover, we

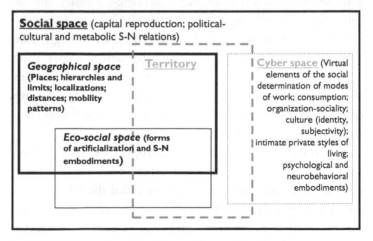

Figure 3.3 Cyberspace and territory as forms of social space.

have clarified some of these forms, distinguishing the *geographical space*—which takes account of places, hierarchies, and limits; localizations; and distances and mobility patterns—from the *ecosocial space*—which encompasses forms of artificialization and socionatural embodiments. In that context, the *territory* appears as a spatial–temporal "cutout" that society as a whole, or some of its peoples, generates as part of its complex social space, where geographical, ecosocial, and cyber processes intertwine. The territory is delimited and shaped when people define a sector of social space as a place for their realization and consolidation as social participants; when they delimit a sufficient and adequate location for their integral social reproduction—that is, the economic, metabolic, cultural, and political reproduction at a particular historical moment, in accordance with strategic collective goals defined through a complex process of social class–gender and ethnic negotiation whose aim is a sustainable, sovereign, solidary, and safe (bio-safe) mode of living.

However, we must also look at the cyberspace through epidemiological eyes, given that its virtual cybernetic processes clearly form part of the social determination of our wellness and healthiness. The 21st-century cyber world, as explained previously, represents the new space of extractivism and a new form of subsumption and social determination of life.

Subsumption, as previously discussed, is determinant of our modes of living. We therefore incorporated it as a crucial category of social determination. What we have called the *fifth subsumption* is nothing more than a complex, accelerated combination of the four previous forms of subsumption. As Karl Marx revealed, during the 16th century *formal subsumption* of work appeared in early manufacturing, and later, during 18th-century industrial revolution, with the advent of mechanization of work, a real, complete labor subsumption came into being. Throughout the second half of the 20th century, scientists working in the biological (e.g., Levins and Lewontin) and health sciences published many texts on social–biological (psychological) subsumption (e.g., Breilh, Laurell-Noriega, and Samaja). In the 21st century, social scientists have also applied the notion to consumption (e.g., Barreda and Veraza). In 2015, I proposed the notion of cybernetic subsumption.

I will not recapitulate my previous arguments on this issue. With the marvelous instruments of the internet and the inauguration of a new era of industry, information and communication are now saddled with the same domination and threats that negatively affect general social life and create inequality. Suffice it to say that the following are worrying examples that raise new questions about public health and prevention: digital platform extractivism, commerce, and labor transformation; massive appropriation and commodification of personal and intimate data; utilization of personal records without consent; the involuntary or "unconscious" proletarianization of everyday life and consumption on Instagram and Facebook; extreme digital penetration and control of our styles of living, behaviors, and political decisions; and the rampant and irresponsible application of artificial intelligence algorithms and artificial biology in the development of robotized social activities and the profitable artificialization of natural life.

This vertiginous movement unleashed by and in the hands of greedy entrepreneurs requires not only a new reading of reality, a rethinking of human life and health and its social determination, but also a new conception of collective and public health actions.

And this entails the need for new categories and analyses and renewed challenges for critical epidemiology.

Critical Epidemiology in Action: The Common Good and the People's Awakening

Critical Epidemiology and the People's Health is a book about the methods and practical role of a challenging academic work indispensable in confronting the serious health problems of an ailing civilization. However, to become a consistent plea for a healthier world, it must propose not only a straightforward assessment and alternative ways of thinking about pivotal problems but also new conceptions of practice for our collective and public health areas. We need to look beyond the technocratic upgrading of conventional practices.

Virchow's (1848) inspiring plea for "full and unlimited democracy" and "radical measures" rather than "mere palliatives" is a powerful call to epidemiologists and health activists. It is also true that, as my dear friend Boaventura Santos, a renowned Portuguese critical epistemologist, has argued, "radical ideas are not directly translated into radical practices and vice versa. . . . This double opacity . . . [occurs because] . . . the established powers today have efficient means with which to prevent the encounter" (B. Santos, 2014). We must therefore promote alternative spaces and action strategies that will allow the meeting of new ideas and forms of agency. To overcome this opacity, a most effective way to connect critical thinking with contesting practices in Latin America has been to recognize the fundamental role of the people in the health system's renovation (León, Jiménez, Vidal, Bermúdez, & De Vos, 2020).

In addition, as has been asserted in the previous chapters, in order to cope with the critical collective health demands of 21st-century societies, it is imperative to not only reform the conceptual basis of health protection, prevention, and promotion, instituting new, effective pathways for transforming our practice, but also consolidate a significant place in science for the people's wisdom and agency.

I have highlighted some major components of the global crisis that are having an impact on our civilization and that hinder healthy living. The basis of this calamity is the fact that "economic inequality is out of control," as Oxfam's *Time to Care* report boldly signals (Coffey et al., 2020). Many health professionals do perceive the evident signs of the regressive trend that is affecting humanity, but they do not always decipher its relation with the uncontrollable indolence of big business and condescending political blindness. Many organized groups want to demolish the patriarchal and colonial pillars of our present societies, but for political and communicational reasons, their voices and powerful arguments frequently do not achieve the indispensable and sustainable political momentum. Nevertheless, people become stronger and enlightened in times of extreme predicament. Social protest has gone beyond the important but limited thrust of unionism. Women and representatives of gender minorities are shaking the foundations of our misogynist and sexist societies. The indigenous national and international confederations are forming cracks in the walls of racism. Conscientious millennial and postmillennial youth are in the streets demanding a stop to the corporations that base their shameful profit rates on the reproduction of inequity and human and natural destruction.

At the current pace, the anthropocentric and fossil fuel-based productive matrix will leave us all without a planet to live on. It is a monstrous cogwheel that moves an inequity-generating machinery, nurtured by intensive oil and coal burning, ~~and~~ making things worse by increasing uncontrolled industrial waste through the intentional planning of product obsolescence. Despite many and severe restraints imposed by the system, conscious 21st-century scientists have struggled for almost two decades to reveal the impacts of this colossal offense, but their studies do not always reveal the perpetrators and ultimate beneficiaries of the capital concentration machinery.

The critical social and life disciplines therefore have no time to waste. In perilous times, the type of functional approach to health science we have extensively critiqued throughout these pages is of limited use. Moreover, often it develops as a counterproductive distractor. Unfortunately, the limited scientific awareness expressed in conventional literature only points at disperse epidemiological indicators, devoid of their historical structural roots and divorced from sustainable collective mobilization.

Empirical studies of climate warming health impacts are a clear example of this type of "forensic" science, which focuses exclusively on dissecting the final life-threatening impacts of criminal industries and their deadly, terminal pathways. Unfortunately, although rigorous and sophisticated climate change studies have generated global concern about those terminal consequences, their limited scope only contributes to incomplete public awareness. They clearly show dramatic tip-of-the-iceberg evidence without signaling those responsible—that is, without tracing the problem's social determination. These days, the outbreak of a pneumonia epidemic in Wuhan City (Hubei, China) triggered by a new family of coronavirus (coronavirus disease 2019), repeats a similar pattern of events. World alarm is created around the problem, focusing exclusively on the unfortunate final outcome of the appearance of a new viral family, without any concern about the social determination of this outcome. This surface-level conceptual framework and practical strategy leaves untouched the need to carefully explore the role of uncontrolled, badly managed animal breeding operations such as the giant hog farms related to the outburst of AH1N1 virus in Mexico (Pew Commission on Industrial Farm Animal Production, 2008), but it also constitutes a dramatic proof of the regrettable divorce between sophisticated conventional biologically centered science (i.e., conventional epidemiology and virology) and solid critical epidemiology. If that unfortunate divide did not exist, the life sciences would have been much more effective in defining opportune socially based prevention. The theory and practice of emergent and re-emergent transmissible processes would have superseded the present empiricist ineffective schemes, the conceptual and technical design of prevention and reparation would focus on the dramatic ecosystem deterioration that multiplies transmission and infectiousness, and the enhanced exposure and transmission patterns at work would have been revealed. In addition, there would have been genome segment expansion and an increased probability of gene recombination in industrial animal farm production and massive animal breeding sites, corresponding transmission acceleration and increasing iRo indexes, reduced animal vulnerability, simple and multiple drug-resistance increases in those contexts, and the unhealthy conversion of previously innocuous social–cultural behaviors and mobilization.

Here, again, the questions are the following: What can the participant health sciences and collective health institutions do to enhance the effectiveness and awareness of social mobilization that demands significant prevention and life-protecting policies? How do we engage in our epidemiological practice for it to become a lever for transformative socially efficient knowledge?

The technical sophistication of research and practice is not enough if science and its institutions are to function in ways contrary to the urgent needs of the people, viewing the world from the privileged standpoint of their own ivory tower. The undeniable advance of biosciences is not enough if our interpretations are trapped in reductionist, abstract, imprecise notions and our agency is self-limited. Let us refer once again to the global problem of unrestrained climate change. If we insist on describing worsening climatic conditions by means of imprecise qualifiers such as "anthropogenic" or on emphasizing terminal facts (e.g., destructive gas accumulation), we would not only be concealing the specific underlying processes of big business negligence but also be giving people misleading evidence and become unwitting accomplices of incomplete social awareness. Most conventional climate research provides robust evidence and brings to the surface the precise and alarming symptoms of oceanic, atmospheric, and terrestrial deterioration, but it is not consistently structured to explain the inherent relations between climatic phenomena and the corporate transgressions that generate them. Fossil fuel production is effectively accused, but we forget that this is merely one link in the chain of the extractivist model at the basis of our ailing civilization. If we keep blaming viral forms of respiratory disease exclusively on viruses strains and vectors, we will be reproducing this same rationale. Organized women, gender, and ethnic minorities are positioning their important claims, but if their claims are isolated, they lose real sustainable and effective political momentum.

Faced with all these radical commitments, critical intercultural science provides an ethical and effective pathway for academic work on our ill planet. That is why understanding the intricacy of life menaces and the congruent development of radical prevention is this book's *leitmotifs*. To affirm our contribution to this ambitious task, in Chapter 1 we provided the reader with a panoramic perspective of the complexity of this global collective health crisis and the greedy economic system that fuels the fire, and we examined the historic construction of Latin American critical collective health as a counteractive force associated with the people's movement. In Chapter 2, we summarized a coherent conceptual critique and methodological alternative with which to confront the flaws and knowledge illusion of hegemonic positivist epidemiology. In doing so, we tied this analysis to the logic and observational changes indispensible for putting epidemiology back on the track of its historical context, liberating it from an imposed Cartesian straightjacket. And now, to follow our line of thinking, in this third chapter we profile some alternative ideas for action.

The earth's health and environmental downfall demand an urgent and productive cooperation among scientists and the people. Unfortunately, we often work in closed circles and rarely incorporate the voice and wisdom of affected communities in our academic reflections about collective health and planning. Most specialists work feverishly to tackle complex problems, but they operate in the potent but limited logic of their own specialty. They often arrive at astounding and valuable findings, and they sincerely think that it is from that narrow perspective that it is possible to build integral solutions. Socially determined individualism and hyperspecialism penetrate universities and research institutions, reproducing a unilateral academic subject.

Meta-Critique of Our Social System: Transdisciplinary and Intercultural Transformative Reasoning

The roots of functional, monomethodic, monocultural, and "Eurocentric" thinking and practice can be found in the long process that began in colonial times. From our perspective, dominant Eurocentric knowledge does not fundamentally refer to the geographical or cultural origin in itself but, rather, to the dominant ontologies and epistemologies contained in the conservative science that accompanied the expansion of European rule, and the racist, patriarchal, and aristocratic philosophies of the ruling groups.[6] As explained previously, in the social and life sciences in particular, the functionally dominant paradigm was *analytic empiricism* (see Chapter 2) in its two main forms of

---

6. We have previously explained that conscientious European thinkers generated crucial contributions to critical, emancipatory science and specifically to critical epidemiology. Therefore, agreement with this complaint and words of caution should not imply that those of us, the supposed "literati" of science, who want to avoid vanguardism must become a rearguard that simply accompanies the creative power and sovereign advance of the supposed "illiterate" from "below" and does not "coopt" them, so as not to contaminate them with Eurocentric or nonnative elements.

inductive methodology: positivist and neo-positivist science in all its different forms and the conservative functional expressions of grounded theory. By applying either quantitative or qualitative reductionism, these scientific paradigms became, willingly or unwillingly, a functional tool of the dominant heuristics and taxonomies of power.

The peoples of the South, and also those of the North, need to establish a critical epistemological inventory to decolonize the theories, methodological elements, and conceptions that submit our scientific and technical work to the extraneous and unilateral principles of functional empiricism.

As Harvey (2007) has insisted in the case of geographical science, there is an asymmetrical relationship between dominant and subaltern scientific paradigms and their mutual valuation. In our case, mainstream, hegemonic biomedical and public health traditions judged from a Eurocentric perspective are assumed to be the repository of truthful, effective knowledge about health and show an evident disinterest in any critical academic counterpart. They also discount important knowledge and thinking that derives from other cultures. Conversely, the critical tradition carefully studies the dominant counterpart in order to extract its positive contributions and supersede the linearity and reductionism of its empiricist views. Critical, challenging arguments entail a contesting theoretical framework that integrates what has been ignored, contextualizes what has been systematically marginalized, and provides a scientific foundation for the critique of the undemocratic nature of our societies. The need for transformative, transdisciplinary, and intercultural knowledge is therefore an objective and subjective condition (Breilh, 2004, 2018c).

To perform this ambitious paradigm shift, critical academic work must not only break away from excessive specialism but also supersede the epistemic silencing of the peoples of other cultures. Major critiques have been published by "native" voices calling for a "methodological decolonization," pointing out that "Western" science does more than oblige a closed positivism, because when referring specifically to indigenous peoples it imposes its particular vision of culture, values, and notions of time and space in order to position a hegemonic theory of knowledge and its power relations (Smith, 1999). Those same voices argue that dominant "Western" scientific narrative seeks to impose (1) its pejorative classification of some societies and cultures, (2) its biased way of representing certain realities, (3) its comparative models, and (4) its historical cultural evaluation criteria (Hall, 1992).

Those are powerful arguments against the complications of "vanguardism" and Eurocentric thinking. But it is also true that core elements of critical social knowledge emerged in the midst of the struggle of the European peoples of the 19th century. It was an egalitarian knowledge, which did not endorse placing Europeanism at its center or obstructing the knowledge of the diversity of otherness.

The structural inequality of the new market society that began on the Old Continent centuries ago also presupposed the formation of critical narratives originating in different disciplinary fields. They emerged as powerful concepts that accompanied the construction of a critical explanation of the European industrial society and the modern civilization that was then taking shape. Many of these concepts, which flourished during the 19th and 20th centuries, sprang from the protests of subaltern Europe. And they are still valid tools that comprise the critical patrimony of the people's struggles throughout the world.

What is significant for our present argument is the need to enhance the people's critical competence and their ability to react to and transform society. In terms of required cognizance, all-hands-on-deck philosophy requires the metacritical aptitudes of all central egalitarian participants.

Metacritical analysis entails the convergence of the diverse critical epistemologies represented in all social participants. Each must be willing to integrate a collaborative social platform that recognizes its strategic interests, but at the same time, every group must be willing to recognize other groups' strategic needs as equal to their own. It also presupposes an epistemic mutual recognition and willingness to accept mutual knowledge transfer and the transgression of conventional statements through complementation.

Metacritical analysis is required to compose an integral perspective of the dominant system of social reproduction and the civilization that sustains it. Different critical perspectives can mutually enhance their capacity as transformative knowledge, disengaging it, at the same time, from any form of vanguardism. This complex cognitive movement implies a transdisciplinary and intercultural democratic operation. Metacritical knowledge consequently allows for the equitable definition of problems and solutions among the social participants involved. It implies a non-elitist complementing of strengths and the mutual compensation of weaknesses in order to build concrete, territorialized actions in a social territory. It entails the respectful sharing of wisdom in order to develop better multicultural transdisciplinary heuristics and stronger taxonomies that comprise transformative collectively based knowledge.

A sustainable metacritical transformative knowledge movement, integrated with community, university, democratic local
and national government representatives, presupposes two fundamental cognitive conditions. First, participant social subjects must
possess compatible epistemic "navigational charts" that allow them
to understand, respect, and move comfortably among the distinct
epistemologies of the social subjects involved. Participants must
be capable of articulating their own knowledge with that built
by the others. Second, metacritical reasoning supposes equitable
participation in defining the general intercultural, theoretical
framework and the specific components of an intercultural and
transdisciplinary historical project of transformation. The material pillar of this emancipatory and complementary social movement is the tangible economic, political, and cultural fairness of
the integrated action program. Metacritical knowledge is not the
simple addition or juxtaposition of the explanatory capacities and
the transformative power of different cultures and groups; rather,
it implies a new cognitive dimension—a dialectical surmounting.
I have proposed it in order to clarify notions such as "knowledge
ecology," generated from an adjacent critical epistemology.

Health inequity is the central embodiment of our civilization.
As I have explained in previous publications, the core element that
I developed in order to study it in my epidemiological research
is the *social power concentration matrix*, which considers class,
gender, and ethnocultural inequity components (Breilh, 1991,
1993b, 1996, 1999, 2003a). Emancipatory metacritical thinking
is powerfully nurtured by all three social subjects, but at this point,
and for the purposes of illustration, I am taking into consideration
ethnic interculturality.

The marvel of critical epidemiology is that it represents an integral look at the complexity of health, whose aim is to help protect the integral wellness required for equitable and healthy societies. Its study object encompasses and articulates the multiple dimensions of general society, social particular modes of living, and personal daily processes in order to understand the socially determined forms of corporal and psychological embodiment: a part of those embodiments constitutes what we understand as disease. Critical epidemiology is by definition transdisciplinary. Figure 3.4 shows the multiple dimensions

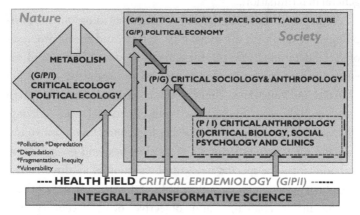

Figure 3.4 Health's complexity and transdisciplinarity (involved disciplinary fields). G, general; I, individual; P, particular.

Breilh, J. (2015a). Epidemiología crítica latinoamericana: Raíces, desarrollos recientes y ruptura metodológica. (La determinación social de la salud como herramienta de ruptura hacia la nueva salud pública—Salud Colectiva). In *Tras las huellas de la determinación* (Memorias de Seminario Inter-universitario de determinación social de la salud; pp. 19–75). Bogotá, Columbia: Universidad Nacional de Colombia.

of social determination of health and highlights the main corresponding academic disciplinary fields of critical science involved in the study of different health domains. This knowledge architecture now must develop dialectically with intercultural knowledge building.

On a general level, the critical theory of space, society, and culture, together with political economy, deals with the processes of social reproduction by capital accumulation, its spatial elements, and general political and cultural relations. Critical and political ecology as disciplines that study the metabolic movement at specific places of society also participate in the understanding of general determination.

At the particular level, the aim of critical sociology and anthropology is to deal with the social class, gender, and ethnic processes of social determination; the subsequent modes of living; and the embodiment of patterns of exposure and vulnerability.

At the individual level, the objective of critical anthropology is to understand the determinant movement of personal styles of living, whereas critical biology, social psychology, and clinics aim to understand the terminal pathways of physiological and psychological embodiments. The specific fields of observation of all three critical disciplinary groups maintain close links with processes of the others.

The major challenge and objective of 21st-century epidemiological knowledge is the construction of participative interdisciplinary–intercultural knowledge platforms. This is widely accepted in contemporary social science departments but is commonly neglected or misinterpreted in conventional public health and epidemiology units. It is useful to briefly discuss this important methodological challenge.

In our previous work, we have highlighted the need to transform the *subject of knowledge* from a unicultural, ivory tower, dominant notion of the academic subject—limited to entitled possessors of a scientifically valid knowledge—to an intercultural, socially based intersubjective notion.[7] This position by no means disdains sound, rigorous, specialized operations as a precondition of scientific knowledge. On the contrary, its objective is to fortify not only the subjective power of transformative knowledge but also, most important, the methodological renewal, enhanced objectivity, and completeness required in critical science.

What Is Real Transdisciplinary Thinking?

A common vagueness or, indeed, straightforward confusion becomes evident when the academic lexicon and meanings assigned to concepts such as *multi*disciplinarity, *inter*disciplinarity, and *trans*disciplinarity are closely examined. As part of ar67 comprehensive publication on this problem, Julie Thompson (2010) provides a clarifying taxonomy. It not only distinguishes the semantic differences between these concepts but also straightforwardly explains the progression of complex knowledge that ranges from the more basic forms of juxtaposition, sequencing, and coordinating included in the concept of multidisciplinarity to the

---

7. Meta-critical knowledge involves emblematic groups of society that represent the strategic emphasis of an articulated program for agency: unions that deal with productive and worker rights; feminist and gender organizations that emphasize gender rights; ethnic organizations that deal with ethnic rights, relationships, and the right to plurinationality and interculturality; ecological organizations that deal with the rights of nature and social–natural metabolism; and health worker and consumer organizations that deal with specific health rights.

more advanced integration, interaction, and blending implied in the concept of interdisciplinarity and the maximum complementation, integration, and collaboration involved in the concept of transdisciplinarity that transcends and transgresses isolated disciplinary work.

In practical terms, and bringing this discussion into the epidemiological field, it is important to realize that transdisciplinary work, by means of careful conceptual and methodological complementation, integration, and collaboration, results in a whole new alternative way of knowing. This respectful approach to other disciplines and the constructive unprejudiced integration of their potentialities makes possible a type of sapient, penetrating, and motivating cognition that exceeds the valuable but incomplete contributions of isolated specialized disciplines, transcending their unidisciplinary boundaries and making possible transformative knowledge.

Intercultural Thinking: Beyond Folkloric Multicultural Affinities

As stated in the introductory notes to this book, the aim is to advance transformative ideas and new ethical standpoints for our practice. A new approach to subvert the philosophy and practice of prevention and promotion is indispensable. A renewed conception of agency is necessary to move from a passive, vertical, bureaucratic agency and surveillance to an active, community-based, accountable, and diversified health action and monitoring movement.

It is crucial to understand that intercultural knowledge goes beyond folkloric multicultural affinities and the mere coexistence of diverse peoples. There exists an ample literature related to critical interculturality that consistently affirms the need to overcome cultural relativism. In the health field, this approach is especially important because, as stated previously, it questions the disengagement of the personal cultural narratives or qualitative evidences from their social relations, and the alienating power of education and the media.

Latin American history provides interesting clues about the profound implications of empowered critical interculturality in health knowledge building. Let us review an illustrative example.

The June 1990 Inti Raymi uprising of the National Confederation of Indigenous Peoples of Ecuador and the eruption of the Zapatista Army of National Liberation (EZLN) in Mexico on January 1, 1994, marked a historical before and after in the Mesoamerican territories of Central and South America. The voice of the native peoples, quenched by colonialism, was heard once again in our painful neoliberal geography. It basically said, "Enough! No more history without us . . . without our dreams, our utopias, our justice and thought."

In claiming their evident right to empower themselves in their culture, principles, rights, and ways of living, they not only emancipated themselves as peoples but also injected an invigorating thrust of energy into the conscience of all humankind. Even in the academic world, the progressive intelligentsia of the academic world was shaken, not for having lacked consciousness of the importance of the indigenous in our vigorous pluriculturalism—indeed, it had provided throughout the centuries abundant examples in the arts and sciences—but because the ancestral worldviews, far from imprisoning us in the past, oxygenated the philosophical–epistemological horizons and the political project of our societies.

In the past three decades, progressive academics have begun to seriously consider the complementarity between scientific and indigenous knowledge. However, within this framework, contradictory arguments have been presented about the validity of subaltern ways of thinking. Contradictory interpretations formed around the "populist" versus "scientifically valid" labels now represent an interesting general scientific theoretical–methodological debate within the social life and health sciences.

Those who reject or belittle intercultural knowledge incur in the same sort of mistrust through which in earlier times, numeric positivism indeed attempted to shield itself from the important advances of scientific trends that contested its alleged objectivity, supposedly independent of the subject, its socially and historically mediated consciousness and its qualitative heuristics. An example of this type of skepticism manifests with regard to the increasing visibility of indigenous worldviews, as is the case of Andean philosophy. "Pachamamism" started to be seen as a regressive view toward a "retro-revolutionary" philosophy of immobility and nostalgia (Sanchez Parga, 2011). The sacred conception of nature, or rather of Mother Nature or the Kichwa "Pachamama," which includes a superior world of celestial entities or deities in accordance with the Andean Chakana, would purportedly condemn our worldview of life to the immobility of the sacred. It has been argued that endorsing principles such as cyclicality and a return to the past—contained in the indigenous narratives and concretely in Andean "ecosophy" (Easterman, 2006)—would necessarily mean the exposure to an ideology of eternal equilibrium. The notion "return to the past" implies the return to times of freedom, solidarity, and sovereignty.

In our view, this type of questioning is perhaps entrapped by the desire to protect a philosophy of transformation and dialectical movement. Perhaps it is also fed by the incompleteness of forms of intellectual practice far removed from the territories where collective struggles are taking place, and demonstrating the transformative anti-establishment sense of indigenous philosophy. Probably it responds to not having been originated in the tangible arena of the defense of life, which is where the wealth of counterhegemonic thought and wisdom of the Andean peoples is to be most directly and powerfully experienced. In one way or another, those negative perspectives on intercultural knowledge lack the epistemic conditions required to understand it, in its profound emancipatory context and breadth.

Popular knowledge is that "which subaltern groups produce and preserve when they control the meaning of their production . . . [incorporate] . . . signs and symbols, senses and meanings, interpretations and semantizations, connotations and denotations, and is subject to the contradictions of the entire context of social production" (Guerra, 1999, p. 60). It embodies innovative elements concerning ways of being, living, and being in a territory that are effective in integrating the metacritical knowledge of society and in building an academic knowledge that breaks with the hegemonic, linear, and reductionist mold.

In the realm of epidemiology, there is currently much writing—although not sufficient—about indigenous thought and its relation to critical academic knowledge. A magnificent recent doctoral dissertation addresses the social determination of health problems in the communities that form the Tucayta organization (i.e., Tukuy Cañaris Ayllukunapak Tantanakuy) of the historic Cañari people in the south of Ecuador (Alulema, 2018). From the perspective of critical epidemiology, it opens the way for an understanding of how a critical academic emancipatory paradigm related to society, life, and health can be complemented by a profound questioning of capitalist society inscribed within the philosophy and the principles—regarding ways of living and nature—of indigenous knowledge. This complement, of which I spoke in a previous essay (Breilh, 2004), was effectively verified in meetings held with organizations of the people at Simon Bolívar Andean University (2007) during the preparatory process leading up to the Constituent Assembly that formulated the new National Constitution of 2008. By working on an intercultural metacritique of rights and the health system, we moved beyond pharma-biomedical reasoning and the reductionism of the old public health, by dialectically integrating the anti-system critique of political economy, critical sociology, and ecology with the principles of plurinationality and the emancipatory interculturality of the people.

Fundamental complementarities were confirmed between our academic concept of healthy modes of living and the indigenous Sumak Kawsay; the questioning of the structure of classist, sexist, and racist inequality and the indigenous philosophy of solidarity, reciprocity, and complementarity; and the notions of the dialectical society–nature metabolism and the principles of relationality of the Andean ecosophy. At the core of both perspectives lies what Ariruma Kowii (2011) describes as Sumak Kawsay's vital, ethical, spiritual, and aesthetic sense of place—of space as a place of life and healing that clashes with the pragmatic mercantile vision of life and wellness. During a recent intercultural workshop, an important distinction was made between two interdependent notions of the indigenous good living: the previously mentioned *sumak kawsay*, which states the general principles and imaginary of wellness, and *alli kawsay*, which defines the practical personal–familiar quotidian, harmonious, creative, and just daily lifestyles (Table 3.1).

Rather than asking whether indigenous knowledge is science or wisdom, rather than using a positivist magnifying glass in order to question and compare knowledge of an intuitive heuristic character and submit it to the analysis of a linear method of empirical correspondence and the experimental reason, and rather than pigeonholing ourselves in a Cartesian perspective in order to demonstrate the supposed inconsistencies of popular knowledge that would not be demonstrable and measurable, we must seriously consider humanity's need to supersede the predominant fragmenting logic. The epistemologically and instrumentally correct questions should then be: How much cognitive and practical value do intercultural perception and knowledge have, and how do we conceive of this value? How much will natural life and human wellness benefit if we overturn the uncontrolled greed contained in the pseudo-philosophy of big business think tanks and substitute it with a cosmovision of the holistic and harmonious development of all forms of life on the planet? What is the value of the sentient-thinking method with which the Andean communities have sustained for centuries the protection of the goods of life and how does it compare with the devastating results of dominant production and its "hard science"? How did indigenous wisdom take care of Mother Nature for centuries while the positivist high-tech green revolution is extinguishing planetary life? How much

Table 3.1 Complementarities of Critical Academic and Indigenous
Thinking

Critical Academic Thinking in Social and Life Sciences	Complex Critical Indigenous Thinking
SOCIAL POLITICAL PHILOSOPHY	
Critique of class, sexist, racist inequality	Philosophy of solidarity, reciprocity, and complementation Decolonization Dynamic and not lineal progress Complementarity and not competence
Ecosocial Philosophy	
Critique of the dialectic deteriorating society–nature metabolism	Principles of ecosophic relationality The harmonious complexity of universe ("Chakana"); the dialects of masculine/feminine, before/after, big/small, superior/inferior; Andean cosmovision
CRITICAL GEOGRAPHY	
Critique of collectively determined and determinant inequitable social space Dominant forms of space support and reproduce dominant forms of social reproduction Savage urbanism (neoliberal city) and rural destructive acceleration Space diversity: social, ecosocial, geographical, and cybernetic	No separation of humans and nature Dynamic changing harmony of the whole's parts The productive space ("Chakra") is the knot around which the community ("Ayllu") weaves social life Chakra is for feeding and not using Mother Nature Chakra is a space for generated and regenerating all forms of life

Table 3.1 **Continued**

Critical Academic Thinking in Social and Life Sciences	Complex Critical Indigenous Thinking
CRITICAL EPIDEMIOLOGY	
Wellness/healthy modes of living Critique of socially determined and segregated modes of living and individual styles of living that constitute contradictory work, consumption, organization, cultural, and metabolic patterns Socially determined collective and individual embodiments, resulting from the clash of collective and individual protective/healthy/wellness versus deteriorating/unhealthy/illness Contradictory development of protective and destructive dimensions of class–gender–ethnically determined social patterns	Sumak Kawsay ("living god") Plentiful, inclusive, harmonious, sublime, collectively protective solidarity, sharing, pleasurable, decolonized, equitable in gender and cultural relations Convivence and plentiful relationship Communitary logic, ecosophic life cosmovision

power do the principles of reciprocity, correspondence, complementarity, and ways of living of an Andean communitarianism have to forge democracy and equity, at a time when the structure and philosophy of economic progress that concentrates wealth and excludes society expand increasingly in unfair and unhealthy spaces and forms of life? In the final reckoning, what is the importance of the solid practical observation of the convincing potential for sustainability and equity of the new way of living that we propose, based on popular knowledge, at a time when all species and our planet, bursting with productive and military technology, are on the verge of collapse?

When we scientists immerse ourselves in natural and social life and distance ourselves from the ideas of an arrogant scientism, we discover—as it has happened in the case of critical epidemiology—that intercultural construction breathes life into an effective metacritique. And in addition to cognitive advances, the willingness to look at ourselves and listen to the affected social subjects, while urged on by transformational knowledge, leads to an intercultural communicative leap forward (Briggs, 2005).

A favorable epistemic effect of adhering to metacritical knowledge is that it elevates methodological consistency and enhances, or even transforms, our capacity as researchers. Building a metacritical outlook depends on articulating the heuristic capacity of different disciplines (transdisciplinarity) and of various cultures (interculturality) in a process of equal competence.

Subverting the Notions of Health Prevention and Promotion

The critique of conventional preventive medicine has been present in Latin America for a long time. In 1972, the publication of *Medical Education in Latin America* by Juan Cesar

García brought about a clear divide between the conservative and functionalist approach of the hegemonic medicine schools and what would become the Latin American movement of social medicine. García proclaimed the need to disengage prevention from the conventional clinical settings. In 1975, the book *The Preventivist Dilemma* by Sergio Arouca—a leading figure of health reform in Brazil—also presented a pioneering critique of preventive medicine. Professor Guillerme Rodríguez, an outstanding early figure of the contemporary Latin American social medicine movement, highlighted the "emergence of a preventive discourse that privileged a new attitude, questioning medical specialism and projecting its practice into the social arena" (Arouca, 1975).

The health field has always been medicalized and converted into an ideal setup for the commercialization of medicine and the reproduction of the farmo-biomedical model. Commonsense notions and biomedical acculturation tend to reproduce the erroneous belief that health is essentially an individual, biopsychological phenomenon that fundamentally depends on personal health care.

As the main beneficiaries of this belief, the biomedical industries make enormous communicative investments in an effort to indoctrinate populations regarding health care, cosmetic, and fitness product consumption. Under this pressure, allopathic health care dependence becomes part of the typical collective modes of living and culture.

This is certainly a complex scenario, in which building an integral demedicalized health system requires the broad and active participation of honest collective and public health experts to promote a new understanding beyond the limits of individual care. Throughout these pages, we have presented some important ideas about how to expand our focus through complex reasoning related to the social determination of health. Opening our minds to the social processes that generate the individual physical (i.e., phenotypical and genetical) and psychological embodiments helps us redefine and extend key notions such as health prevention and promotion (Figure 3.5).

Conventional medicalized prevention is limited to individual health care spaces, with certain incursions into the domain of

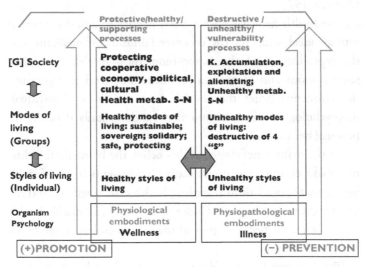

	Protective/healthy/ supporting processes	Destructive / unhealthy/ vulnerability processes
[G] Society	**Protecting cooperative economy, political, cultural Health metab. S-N**	**K. Accumulation, exploitation and alienating; Unhealthy metab. S-N**
Modes of living (Groups)	**Healthy modes of living: sustainable; sovereign; solidary; safe, protecting**	**Unhealthy modes of living: destructive of 4 "S"**
Styles of living (Individual)	**Healthy styles of living**	**Unhealthy styles of living**
Organism Psychology	Physiological embodiments **Wellness**	Physiopathological embodiments **Illness**

(+)PROMOTION   (−) PREVENTION

Figure 3.5 Prevention and promotion redefined: the multidimensional epidemiological profile (Breilh, 1977, 2003a, 2015a).

familial domestic styles of living. This conventional model at best projects prevention to what Leavell and Clark (1965) define as primary, secondary, and tertiary prevention, according to a triadic configuration of ecological prevention (i.e., host, agent, and environment). This refers to *primary prevention* in the prepathogenic stage when the agent can come in contact with the host and early prevention and health promotion measures can be taken; *secondary prevention* in the beginning of the pathogenic stage, when early diagnosis and timely health care can impede the problem from advancing and provoking the person's disability; and *tertiary prevention*, which refers to the rehabilitation that stops the disabling process of disease (Leavell & Clark, 1965). The model promotes interesting actions but still limited to the terminal period of epidemiological determination and to the individual domain. Our critical epidemiology model implies actions not only at this level of individual prevention but also, fundamentally, those identified in the multidimensional profile.

The transforming concepts about health prevention and promotion, running parallel to the advances of the social and biological sciences, are breaking the limits of conventional public health. The interdependent relationship between the arts and health is one fascinating case of transdisciplinarity. Current research is proof of the visionary outlook of Henry Sigerist (1944), who clearly proclaimed its importance in the development of a healthy civilization. The case of music, for instance, not only makes that relation evident but also demonstrates that it can be subject to differing interpretations. Maria Cristina Breilh (2019) notes that the most frequent interpretation has considered music's therapeutic value in individuals—a tradition based on neuroscientific research—but, conversely, insists on music's role as a potent element of modes of living and its influence on the collective wellness/healthy living.

In all our research and teaching projects using the critical processes matrix, we have systematized the various multidomain actions of what we have called *deep prevention*.[8] To exemplify this, in our project on the social determination of dengue, we included in the preventive scheme organized around the respective critical process matrix with its different embodiments all the generating elements throughout the three dimensions. At the general level, we consider actions that deteriorate ecosystems and the territorial metabolism, flooding the environment with pesticides and destroying the entomological vector–predator balance; policies and regional plans that allow and promote the destruction of territorial biodiversity, exacerbate climate warming, and foster neoliberal city development and inequitable spatial segregation; and policies that widen the social disparity of vulnerable urban populations. We have also included conditions at the particular level, such as typically social class segregated patterns of vector breeding spaces, human exposure, and vulnerability patterns. Finally, also included are socially determined conditions and embodiments in individuals and their families that develop under the heavy influence of the general and particular realities but can be seen in concrete household exposure embodiments, personal vulnerabilities, and forms of viral inoculation.

---

8. Deep or profound prevention penetrates all domains of the multidimensional epidemiologic profile (see Figure 3.5) and takes into account all the nodes of the respective critical process matrix.

The Importance of Transforming Epidemiological Surveillance: Reinforcing the Precautionary Principle and the "Triangle of Action"

Conventional epidemiological surveillance suffers from the same shortcomings we have been examining. It was designed as a component of the biomedical logic of health services.

Conventional epidemiological surveillance is focused on individual disease, operates on isolated risk factors, is vertical and state centered, annuls the real participation and social intelligence of communities, and is inefficient and expensive. In order to harmonize this tool with our proposed model, Table 3.2 shows the main transformations to be made in order to build what we have designated as participative, community-based, critical strategic health monitoring (Breilh, 2003b).

Epidemiological caution is fundamental for the protection of life and the recovery of rights presupposed by healthy living. As explained previously, the precautionary principle states that if there is reasonable suspicion that a process could be harmful to human life and health, if there is scientific uncertainty about its harmfulness, then there exists an ethical duty and responsibility to take action. In that case, we must proceed by transferring the burden of proof from the community that suffers the problem to those whose activities are causing it, through a transparent, informed, and democratic decision-making process that includes those affected.

Table 3.2 Conventional Health Surveillance Versus Strategic Participative Health Monitoring

Dimension	Conventional Epidemiological Surveillance	Strategic Participative Monitoring
Object	Disease (cases); individual illness expressions; health public care actions	Collective health; critical processes (protective and destructive); respective embodiments
Concepts/ theoretical fundaments	Causality; large-scale public etiological prevention	Social determination of health (collective and individual); complex thinking—critical epidemiology; strategic planning, social control, and participative accountability
Social subjects	State-centered decision-makers; centralized vertical health intelligence	Public state and social conduction; participative health intelligence bodies; social–community organizations under cooperation with intersectoral public decision-makers
Type of participation	Passive, collaborative "lay reporting"	Participative empowering two-way health intelligence
Information system/ organization	Vertical; centralized; inefficient; expensive; limited coverage; centripetal information flow	Strategic political logic focused on the peoples' interest; three subsystems: critical monitoring, immediate reaction, communication participation

Precautionary action should not be limited to focusing on the terminal stages of identified problems, when destructive processes have already generated deleterious consequences. Its importance as a preventive and health rights tool is so great that the social organizations of Ecuador and our university fought to incorporate it into the Constitution of 2008. After interminable debate, it was finally consecrated in the 32nd article of the Constitution's second chapter, which institutes "the right to good living," whereby it is assumed as a fundamental principle of public health rights.

Having briefly profiled throughout this chapter some proposals for transforming the logic of epidemiological reasoning—as viewed from a critical academic perspective—it is important to articulate our renewed thinking to a new conception of health planning and incidence contained in theory "*policy triangle*" and its implications for emancipatory scientific intercultural transdisciplinary articulation of critical research, graduate teaching, and policy incidence networking strategies (Matus, 1987). Alternative networking that links transformative thinking and mobilized communities and scientific–instrumental resources requires (1) an emancipatory project for health (critical health theory project and strategic impact project on the critical processes of social determination), (2) an articulated social block of affected communities and concerned and mobilized stakeholders, and (3) a body of scientific knowledge and useful technical tools redesigned to fit the needs of the two prior elements.

If the guiding canons of a democratic inclusive 21st-century collective health science are intercultural and transdisciplinary, then the field of critical epidemiology comprises not just specialized epidemiology and academic membership. Our main challenge in this new century is to embed within our theory and method valid and potent heuristic and taxonomical elements successfully developed in non-"Western" knowledge. Even in the most specialized issues or problems, we enrich and strengthen our thoughts and methods by integrating and complementing our academic tools with sophisticated ideas and resources developed in other cultural and social settings. Euro-USA-centric prejudicial thinking attempts to persuade us that academia is the exclusive space for thought and action—the only singing voice and discerning mind.

This democratization and decolonization of science by no means implies our neglect or underestimation of scientific rigor (Breilh et al., 2012). Hence, we have insisted on the need to consolidate a renewed perspective with regard to the role of universities and research centers. Five cardinal academic tasks profile the role of the critical collective health academic and research programs: (1) promotion of holistic knowledge and critical research; (2) development of technical instruments to enable changes with the objective of a healthy life; (3) advancement of tools for the social control, oversight, and accountability of policymakers and management; (4) consolidation of intercultural and interdisciplinary construction mechanisms for research/advocacy; and (5) their contribution to democratic community-based empowerment.

The Challenge of Rethinking 21st-Century Universities

The primordial role of universities and the problems of humanity cannot be understood and evaluated today without considering the present crisis of our societies. Universities are one important source of informed consciousness.

We witness the striking advances of science and technology while at the same time the most painful and highest levels of decomposition of real conditions for social reproduction on the planet (Arizmendi, 2007).

We must put an end to the rampant growth of a biased science by contract that cannot withstand any serious ethical assessment of its conflicts of interest. Big money is twisting our arms, stealing our souls, reproducing the "sins of experts" in project evaluators and curricular accreditation. Corporate pressure and direct ownership of academic institutions and research centers are deviating our work from the most urgent problems by introducing their profit priorities.

In the health field, the biomedical bubble that we have described previously is neutralizing critical academic assessment of the decadence of our well-being. Universities, being the fundamental source of independent critical thinking, have the responsibility to defend transformative knowledge and to underpin social empowerment and contribute with academic excellence to a much-needed social reform.

Academic autonomy and scholarly reform naturally depend on the historical condition and context. And that context is the promising, but at the same time threatening, society of the 21st century. We must protect our universities from turning into diligent branches of companies that assume scientific knowledge as an instrument of profit rather than a means to solve the grave problems of humanity.

An alert academy is needed, open and deeply connected to people and rooted in critical thinking that is capable of facing hegemony supported by functional science. We need to build platforms that link up with people's needs and demands. We need to create efficient relations with conscientious public services. Within this historical framework, universities are the spaces called upon to safeguard self-awareness and thus must overcome functional agendas.

If we want to protect the spirit of unrestricted responsible academic work, our central task is to transform the interpretative models and the logic of explanation that have invaded our programs and syllabi. We must open the doors of our classrooms to our people and open up university spaces to community-based research and teaching. Technical advocacy is also a necessary contribution. We must firmly and peacefully revolutionize academic ethics. The democratization of access to bibliographic resources is imperative and feasible, as demonstrated by the exemplary decision of the University of California to reallocate its bulky journal subscriptions budget from an expensive privatized to open access journal system (Fox & Brainard, 2019). Faculties and schools that work with life sciences (i.e., faculties of health sciences, agricultural sciences, biology, biochemistry, etc.) as well as humanities and social, cultural, and political sciences, which deal with vital issues such as law, cultural critique, social organization, and power structures, must use consistent tools to unravel the threats they know impact life. We must break the vicious cycle of studies undertaken with goodwill but imbued with functional models, tools, and data.

The severity of the current global crisis naturally offers violent strategies as a false way out. There is desperation in the face of the obscene multiplication of a decadent, opulent, and rapacious behavior of the "world's 2,153 billionaires ... [who] ... have more wealth than the 4.6 billion people who make up 60% of the planet's population" (Coffey et al., 2020).

Therefore, the reorganization of superior education is one of the urgent actions needed for collective and public health reform. In that spirit, the Health Sciences Area of the most important graduate university of Ecuador (UASB-E) has organized an ambitious transformation of its master's, doctoral, and postdoctoral programs. In the past 10 years, first as dean and more recently as rector (2016–2018), I have witnessed the successful development of groundbreaking research, teaching, and advocacy programs, sustained by the tireless work of dozens of professors and graduate students. Our team is committed to research and advocacy projects with dozens of communities of agricultural, industrial, mining, and garbage recycling workers; indigenous, women's, and consumer organizations; academic communities; health workers; students; adolescents; and many more groups that form part of our research and teaching programs.

In that arduous but rewarding path, interesting transformations of the academic model have been produced and innovative scientific contributions have been made. Our own graduate students— some of whom are now prestigious members of our teaching staff—or those who we receive as visiting scholars from Latin American, North American, or European countries have made significant contributions to the development of participative research.

To briefly characterize some of our current advancements, I highlight four emblematic lines of action. A team led by Fernanda Soliz works on the metabolic and epidemiological impacts of mega-mining (Soliz Torres, 2018) and also focuses on the social determination of the health of informal recyclers and their families who live and work in the open landfill of Canton Portoviejo, Ecuador. The team also works on the political ecology and critical geography of waste, analyzing the distribution of health impacts according to a typology of the recyclers' modes of living in relation to its five dimensions, as defined by our critical epidemiology model, systematizing and adapting the critical participative community-based monitoring model that we proposed (Soliz, 2016).

In 2017, we inaugurated an emblematic inter-institutional participative research and policy incidence program, AndinaEcosaludable. As rector of the institution, I proposed to articulate various projects: (1) the TEG3 research we have developed to support agro-ecological bananas for export production in the southern coastal region of Machala and to provide scientific cooperation in order to explain the social determination of nutrition and the chemical contamination of food for the children of the municipal crèche system (Children Development Centers) of the government of Cayambe—a leading cut flower for export production region—with the valuable collaboration of the University of British Columbia; (2) the Experimental Research and Training System on Agro-ecology and Health (SEICAS), a platform for undergraduate and graduate students and volunteers from both our own and other universities that studies the transition from conventional to agro-ecological agriculture, provides safe food to and in solidarity with urban consumers in Quito, and collaborates with local producers to enhance their agro-ecological capacities; and (3) the solidarity alliance of our program with 12 gender rights communities composed of women agro-ecological producers, for the permanent provision of safe, chemical-free food to our institution's catering services and weekly open fair, integrating at the same time the national movement of agro-ecological advocates that operate around similar fairs.

The program has been consolidated based on the support of our academic community, the current authorities, and important social organizations, but also the scientific and technical contribution of our academic staff. In this process of consolidation, the program design and intercultural relations have received the enthusiastic support of our researchers. Our coordinator, María José Breilh, a specialist in critical health communication, is developing communicative materials and an academic framework for postgraduate training in this field. Ylonka Tillería, after successfully completing our PhD program, participates in coordinating innovative graduate courses and, with Maria José Breilh, Mónica Izurieta, and Doris Guilcamaigua, in our international "science and resistance" radio program. Mónica Izurieta, a doctoral candidate and teacher, is successfully coordinating the SEICAS program, contributing at the same time with her expertise in food consumption systems and the general administration of the program. Giannina Zamora is an accredited leader and scientist of a national critical geography organization, PhD candidate in our doctoral program, and coordinator of the spatial analysis components of our projects. Orlando Felicita, also a doctoral candidate and expert in chromatography, is responsible for the technical coordination of our laboratories and is constructing alternative toxicity evaluation protocols. Doris Guilcamaigua, doctoral candidate, is currently working on the development of a comprehensive ecosystems and human impact evaluation system for agriculture. The junior members of our lab, Stephanie Villamarín and Mayumi Alta, work in the atomic absorption and biomarkers operations dedicated to detecting heavy metals and toxicity in different environmental and human samples. Also, the individual alternative integrative health group, led by José Luís Coba, PhD candidate and well-known expert in Chinese medicine, is studying the contributions of Chinese philosophy to the understanding of the social determination of health. Catalina Lopez and Maria Sandoval conduct research and graduate teaching regarding the critical processes of child development.

The conceptual and methodological components require the contribution of our teaching staff. Luiz Allan Kunzle and Maria de Lourdes Larrea contribute their expertise in mathematical model training so useful for our advances in non-Cartesian quantitative analysis. Bayron Torres, our expert programmer and data analyst, provides his skills for innovative data analysis.

Our team's capacities and integration illustrate the conscious, solidary, and collective nature of our Health Area and its trans-disciplinary expertise. Those are two fundamental requisites of transformative multifaceted research collaboration. The program benefits from their valuable contributions in a variety of problems: intercultural activities with our community and institutional partners, diverse lab and analysis sessions, post-graduate teaching, innovative events, and alternative health communication.

This type of cooperation is possible in democratic academic settings, in which the search for scientific excellence and responsible contribution is free from the arrogance and unhealthy competitiveness that sometimes cloud reason and inhibit comradeship.

Writing this book has reaffirmed my conviction that critical epidemiology needs to link the potent valuable resources of the peoples from the South and the North. A history of universal inequity has interposed differences that sometimes act as barriers. Only a compassionate standpoint will put us all back on the human track in order to defend our species and a future of authentic wellness. Here are some deeply humane, motivating, and timely voices that demonstrate the long-standing traditions of intercultural philosophy and human wisdom, coming from the South and the North:

Of fire was then our word.
To wake up who slept.
To outrage who was satisfied and surrendered.
To reveal history ... force her to say what was silent. ...
We look for in our ancestral history, in our collective heart. ...
We were building what we are and that not only keeps us alive
    and resisting, but also lifts us worthy and rebellious.
        —EZLN (The war against oblivion General Command
                of Zapatista Army of National Liberation;
            Subcomandantes Insurgentes Moisés y Galeano)

And in this time of coldness, when Earth smells of human dust and is so sad, I would like to knock on all doors, beg whomever for pardon, and make him/her small fresh bread loaves, in the oven of my heart.
        —Cesar Vallejo (The voice of Latin American poet,
                "Los Heraldosnegros," 1918)

A human being is part of the whole, called by us the "Universe," a part limited in time and space. He experiences himself, his thoughts and feelings as something separated from the rest— a kind of optical delusion of his consciousness. This delusion is a kind of prison for us, restricting us to our personal desires and to affection for a few persons nearest to us. Our task must be to free ourselves from this prison by widening our circle of compassion to embrace all living creatures and the whole nature in its beauty. Nobody is able to achieve this completely, but the striving for such achievement is in itself a part of the liberation, and a foundation for inner security.

—Albert Einstein (The voice of a European
scientist, Letter, 1950)

It is generally thought that profound change in a society is achieved exclusively from politics or technology. Notwithstanding, historic studies reveal this ascertainment is fragile. The real and sustainable transformation of a society is fundamentally achieved through a consistent transformation of the peoples' ways of life, the overcoming of cultural barriers and passive functional ideas that sustain conformism—that is, from the way of operating, explaining, imagining, creating, and dreaming about our reality. Politics and technology are rather the instruments that help us move the gears created by social mobilization and our creations at work, culture, and science—in short, by the ways we conduct our lives. The transformation, therefore, does not come exclusively and fundamentally from political and technical ideas but, rather, from the principles and ways of operating and dreaming about a new equitable and healthier civilization.

Within that framework, culture and science are, nevertheless, not reduced to the pure world of generating powerful ideas
but, rather, comprise part of the complex and fascinating world
of material actions guided by consciousness and compassion.
Conscientious ethical changes in the ways of thinking are made
possible in concrete historical periods and are born from transformative ways of doing. Radical ideas that interplay with real
problem-solving movements become a transformative force. All
that to argue that critical science is not reduced to a theoretical set
but, rather, constitutes an embodiment of years of activity, work,
and search, which help us understand the desirable and repudi-
ating aspects of life, giving spiritual oxygen and intellectual thrust
to our people.

REFERENCES

Acero, M. (2010). *Zoonosis, animal health and other public health problems related to animals: Theoretical and methodological reflections.* Doctoral dissertation, Interdisciplinary Doctoral Program on Public Health, National University of Colombia, Bogotá, Colombia.

Acosta, A. (2013). Extractivism and neo-extractivism: Two sides of the same curse. In M. Lang & D. Mokrani (Eds.), *Beyond development: Alternative visions from Latin America* (pp. 61–86). Quito, Ecuador: Fundación Rosa Luxemburg/Abya Yala.

Aguilar, M. (2019, August 14). Salud Pública en shock. *El Comercio.* Retrieved from https://www.elcomercio.com/opinion/salud-publica-shock-marcelo-aguilar.html#.XUl8Po8-7vs.whatsapp

Allende, S. (1939). *La realidad médico-social chilena.* Santiago: Ministerio de Salubridad, Previdencia y Asistencia Social.

Almeida-Filho, N. (2000). *La ciencia tímida: Ensayos de deconstrucción de la epidemiología.* Buenos Aires, Argentina: Lugar Editorial. Retrieved from http://www.casadellibro.com/libro-la-ciencia-timida-ensayos-de-deconstruccion-de-la-epidemiologia/9508920955/881504

Almeida-Filho, N., Pan American Health Organization, & World Health Organization. (1992). Epidemiología sem números: Una introducción crítica a la ciencia epidemiológica. Retrieved from http://www.bvsde.paho.org/documentosdigitales/bvsde/texcom/cd045364/01740.pdf

Alulema, R. (2018). *La sabiduría cañari de la chacra en relación con la salud y el ambiente, frente a la modernización agropecuaria en la organización Tucayta.* Doctoral dissertation, Universidad Andina Simón Bolívar, Quito, Ecuador.

Alvaredo, F., Chancel, L., Piketty, T., Saez, I., & Zucman, G. (2018). *World inequality report 2018.* Berlin, Germany: World Inequality Lab.

Arendt, H. (1968). *Imperialism.* New York, NY: Harcourt Brace Jovanovich.

Arístegui, C. (2019). *Expone Dussel trasfondo de la ideología evangelista para justificar golpes de Estado* [Video]. Retrieved from http://aristeguinoticias.com

Arizmendi, L. (2007). El florecimiento humano como mirador iconoclasta ante la mundialización de la pobreza. *Desacatos: Revista de Ciencias Sociales* (23). Retrieved from https://doi.org/10.29340/23.636

Arouca, S. (1975). *O dilema preventivista. Contribuçao para a comprençao e crítica de medicina preventiva.* Campinas, Brazil: Tesis de doutoramento da Facultad de Ciencias Médicas da UNICAMP.

Aspin, D. N. (1995). Logical empiricism, post-empiricism and education. In P. Higgs (Ed.), *Metatheories in philosophy of education* (pp. 21–49). Johannesburg, South Africa: Heinemann.

Ayres, J. R. (1997). *Sobre o risco: Para compreender a epidemiologia.* São Paulo, Brazil: HUCITEC.

Barata, R., Barreto, M., Almeida-Filho, N., & Veras, R. P. (Eds.). (1997). *Eqüidade e saúde: Contribuições da epidemiologia.* Rio de Janeiro, Brazil: Editora Fiocruz/ABRASCO.

Barreda, A. (2008). *El urbanismo salvaje.* Ponencia en el Foro Social Mundial, Derecho a la ciudad y el hábitat, Mesa "Derecho a la ciudad, el hábitat y a la vivienda," January 23.

Barreto, M. L., De Almeida-Filho, N., & Breilh, J. (2001). Epidemiology is more than discourse: critical thoughts from Latin America. *J Epidemiol Community Health, 55*(3), 158–159.

Bartra, A. (2006). El capital en su laberinto: De la renta de la tierra a la renta de la vida. Universidad Autónoma de la Ciudad de México, Editorial Itaca, CEDRSSA.

Beckfield, J. (2018). *Political Sociology and The People's Health.* New York, NY: Oxford University Press.

Behm, H. (1992). *Desigualdades sociales ante la muerte en América Latina.* Santiago, Chile: CELADE.

Bhaskar, R. (1986). *Scientific realism and human emancipation.* London, UK: Verso.

Birn, A. E., & Muntaner, C. (2019). Latin American social medicine across borders: South-South cooperation and the making of health solidarity. *Glob Public Health, 14*(6–7), 817–834.

Birn A-E, Pillay Y, Holtz TH. *Textbook of Global Health*. 4th ed. New York, NY: Oxford University Press, 2017.

Bijoy, C. (2018). Lessons from Plachimada. In N. C. Narayanan, S. Parasuraman, & R. Ariyabandu (Eds.), *Water governance and civil society responses in South Asia*, pp. 309–342. London, UK: Routledge. doi.org/10.4324/9781315734071

Black, D., & Whitehead, M. (1988). Inequalities in health: The Black report. In P. Townsend & N. Davidson (Eds.), *The health divide*. London, UK: Penguin.

Boltvinik, J. (2005, January). Ampliar la mirada: Un nuevo enfoque de la pobreza y el florecimiento humano. *Papeles de Población, 11*(44).

Bourdieu, P. (1998). *O poder simbólico*. Rio de Janeiro, Brazil: Bertrand Brasil.

Bowker, G. C., & Star, S. L. (1999). *Sorting things out: Classification and its consequences*. Cambridge, MA: MIT Press.

Brauer, F. (2017). Mathematical epidemiology: Past, present, and future. *Infectious Disease Modeling, 2*(2), 113–127. doi:10.1016/j.idm.2017.02.001

Breilh, J. (1977). *Crítica a la interpretación ecológico funcionalista de la epidemiología: Un ensayo de desmitificación del proceso salud enfermedad*. Mexico City, Mexico: Universidad Autónoma Metropolitana de Xochimilco.

Breilh, J. (1979). *Epidemiología: Economía, Medicina y Política* (1st ed.). Quito, Ecuador: Universidad Central del Ecuador.

Breilh, J. (1989). *Breve recopilación sobre operacionalización de la clase social para encuestas en la investigación social*. Quito, Ecuador: Centro de Estudios y Asesoría en Salud. Retrieved from http://hdl.handle.net/10644/3565

Breilh, J. (1991). *La triple carga (Trabajo, práctica doméstica y procreación): Deterioro prematuro de la mujer en el neoliberalismo*. Quito, Ecuador: CEAS.

Breilh, J. (1993a). Trabajo hospitalario, estrés y sufrimiento mental: Salud internos en Quito. *Revista Salud Problema, 23*, 21–38.

Breilh, J. (1993b). *Género, poder y salud.* Quito, Ecuador: Universidad Técnica del Norte/CEAS.

Breilh, J. (1994). Las ciencias de la salud pública en la construcción de una prevención profunda. In M. I. Rodriguez (Ed.), *Lo biológico y lo social: Su articulación en la formación del personal de salud* (Serie Desarrollo de Recursos Humanos, Vol. 101, pp. 63–100). Washington, DC: Pan American Health Organization/World Health Organization. Retrieved from http://hist.library.paho.org/Spanish/DRH/21485.pdf

Breilh, J. (1996). *El género entrefuegos: Inequidad y esperanza.* Quito, Ecuador: CEAS.

Breilh, J. (1997). *Nuevos Conceptos y Técnicas de Investigación* (3rd ed.). Quito, Ecuador: CEAS.

Breilh, J. (1999). La inequidad y la perspectiva de los sin poder: Construcción de lo social y del género. In M. Viveros & G. Garay Ariza (Eds.), *Cuerpo, diferencias y desigualdades: Simposio del VIII Congreso de Antropología en Colombia, Diciembre de 1997* (pp. 130–141). Centro de Estudios Sociales, Facultad de Ciencias Humanas, U. Nacional.

Breilh, J. (2001). *Eugenio: La otra memoria: Nueva lectura de la historia de las ideas científicas.* Cuenca, Ecuador: Universidad de Cuenca, Facultad de Ciencias Médicas: Centro de Estudios y Asesoría en Salud–Consejo Internacional de Salud de los Pueblos.

Breilh, J. (2003a). *Epidemiología crítica ciencia emancipadora e interculturalidad.* Buenos Aires, Argentina: Lugar Editorial.

Breilh, J. (2003b). De la vigilancia convencional al monitoreo participativo. *Ciencia e SaúdeColetiva, 8*(4), 937–951.

Breilh, J. (2004). Epidemiología crítica ciencia emancipadora e interculturalidad (2nd ed.). Buenos Aires, Argentina: Lugar Editorial.

Breilh, J. (2007). New model of accumulation and agro-business: The ecological and epidemiological implications of the Ecuadorian cut flower production. *Ciência & Saúde Coletiva, 12*(1), 91–104. Retrieved from http://www.scielo.br/scielo.php?pid=S1413-81232007000100013&script=sci_arttext

Breilh, J. (2010). *Epidemiología: Economía política y salud* (7th ed.). Quito, Ecuador: Universidad Andina.

Breilh, J. (2011). The subversion of the good life (enlightened rebelliousness for the 21st century: A critical perspective on the work of Bolívar Echeverría). *Salud Colectiva English Edition, 7*(3), 389–397.

Breilh, J. (2013). *Proyecto de investigacion sobre la teoria de la determinacion social de la salud la critica de la nocion del "buen vivir."* Quito, Ecuador: Fondo de Investigacion de la Universidad Andina Simon Bolivar.

Breilh, J. (2015a). Epidemiología crítica latinoamericana: Raíces, desarrollos recientes y ruptura metodológica. (La determinación social de la salud como herramienta de ruptura hacia la nueva salud pública—Salud Colectiva). In *Tras las huellas de la determinación* (Memorias de Seminario Inter-universitario de determinación social de la salud; pp. 19–75). Bogotá, Columbia: Universidad Nacional de Colombia.

Breilh, J. (2015b). Epidemiology of the 21st century and cyberspace: Rethinking power and the social determination of health. *Revista Brasileira de Epidemiologia, 18*(4), 965–975.

Breilh, J. (2016). *Espejo, adelantado de la ciencia crítica (una "antihistoria" de sus ideas en salud).* Quito, Ecuador: Universidad Andina Simón Bolívar y Corporación Editora Nacional.

Breilh, J. (2017a). *Matriz de procesos críticos: fundamentos teórico explicativos.* Quito, Ecuador: Dirección Nacional de Derechos de Autor y Conexos. Certificado: QUI-052531; Trámite: 002302-2017.

Breilh, J. (2017b). *INSOC (Cuestionario para la investigación de la inserción social en la investigación: Fundamentos teóricos y explicativos)* (No. 002301). Quito, Ecuador: Dirección Nacional de Derechos de Autor y Conexos.

Breilh J. (2018a). *Herramientas de la epidemiología crítica para desarrollar el principio de precaución.* Paper presented at the Conferencia al Seminario Internacional "Nuevas Tendencias Tecnológicas y sus Impactos en América Latina," Mexico City, Mexico, May 21.

Breilh, J. (2018b). Contribuciones teórico-metodológicas de la medicina ecuatoriana para la investigación de la inequidad social y la desigualdad en salud. In J. Breilh (Ed.), *La medicina ecuatoriana en el siglo XXI* (Vol. 3, pp. 57–73). Quito, Ecuador: Universidad Andina Simón Bolívar-Corporación Editora Nacional.

Breilh, J. (2018c). Critical epidemiology in Latin America: Roots, philosophical and methodological ruptures. In J. Vallverdú, A. Puyol, & A. Estany (Eds.), *Philosophical and methodological debates in public health* (pp. 21–46) Cham, Switzerland: Springer.

Breilh, J. (2019). *Ciencia crítica sobre impactos en la salud colectiva y ecosistemas (Guía investigativa pedagógica, evaluación de las 4 "S" de la vida).* Quito, Ecuador: Andina EcoSaludable, UASB-E.

Breilh, J., Campaña, A., Hidalgo, F., Sánchez, D., Larrea, M., Felicita, O., . . . López, J. (2005). Floriculture and the health dilemma: Towards fair and ecological flower production. In *Latin American health watch: Alternative Latin American health report.* Quito, Ecuador: CEAS.

Breilh, J., Granda, E., Campaña, A., & Betancourt, O. (1983). *Ciudad y Muerte Infantil: El deterioro de la salud capitalismo.* Quito, Ecuador: Ediciones CEAS.

Breilh, J., Pagliccia, N., & Yassi, A. (2012). Chronic pesticide poisoning from persistent low-dose exposures in Ecuadorean floriculture workers: Toward validating a low-cost test battery. *International Journal of Occupational and Environmental Health, 18*(1), 7–21.

Breilh, J., & Tillería Muñoz, Y. (2009). *Aceleración global y despojo en Ecuador: El retroceso del derecho a la salud en la era neoliberal.* Quito, Ecuador: Universidad Andina Simón Bolívar/Abya Yala.

Breilh, M. C. (2019). *An approximation to the statement of aesthetic value: Examining performance art/studies* [Essay]. University of British Columbia Interdisciplinary Doctoral Program, Vancouver, British Columbia, Canada.

Breilh J. (2019). Critical epidemiology in Latin America: roots philosophical and methodological ruptures. In: Methodological Ruptures. In J. Vallverdú, A. Puyol, A. Estany (Eds.), *Philosophical and Methodological Debates in Public Health.* Springer, Cham. doi:https://doi.org/10.1007/978-3-030-28626-2_3

Breilh J. (2003). *Epidemiología Crítica: Ciencia Emancipadora e Interculturalidad.* Buenos Aires, Argentina; Lugar Editorial, S.A.

Breilh, J. (2008). Latin American critical ("social") epidemiology: new settings for an old dream. *Int J Epidemiol, 37*(4), 745–750.

Briggs, C. (2005). Critical perspectives on health and communicative hegemony: Progressive possibilities, lethal connections. *Revista de Antropología Social, 14*, 101–124.

Briggs, C. L., & Mantini-Briggs, C. (2003). *Stories in the time of cholera: Racial profiling during a medical nightmare.* Berkeley, CA: University of California Press.

Bringsjord, S., & Govindarajulu, N. S. (2018, Fall). Artificial intelligence. In E. N. Zalta (Ed.), *The Stanford encyclopedia of philosophy.* Retrieved from https://plato.stanford.edu/archives/fall2018/entries/artificial-intelligence

Broadbent, A. (2013). *Philosophy of epidemiology.* Houndmills, UK: Palgrave Macmillan.

Bronfman, M. (1992). Infant mortality and crisis in México. *International Journal of Health Services, 22,* 157–168.

Bunge, M. (1972). *Causalidad (El principio de causalidad en la ciencia moderna)* (3rd ed.). Buenos Aires, Argentina: EDEBA.

Cañete, R., et al. (2015). *Privilegios que niegan derechos: Desigualdad extrema y secuestro de la democracia en América Latina y el Caribe.* Oxford, UK: Oxfam.

Carrillo, R. (1951). *Plan sintético de Salud Pública 1952–1958.* Buenos Aires, Argentina: Ministerio de Salud Pública de la Nación.

Casallas, A. L. (2019). *Aportes y desafíos de la salud colectiva latinoamericana una perspectiva histórica* (Tesis doctoral en Salud Colectiva, Ambiente y Sociedad). Universidad Andina Simón Bolívar Sede Ecuador, Quito, Ecuador.

Coffey, C., Espinoza Revollo, P., Harvey, R., Lawson, M., Parvez Butt, A., Piaget, K., . . . Thekkudan, J. (2020). *Time to care: Unpaid and underpaid care work and the global inequality crisis.* Oxford, UK: Oxfam. https://doi.org/10.21201/2020.5419

Cohen, I. B. (1985). *Revolution in science.* Cambridge, MA: Belknap.

Cohen, J. (1994). The earth is round ($p < .05$). *American Psychologist, 49*(12), 997–1003. https://doi.org/10.1037/0003-066X.49.12.997

Cordeiro, J. (2019). *Singularity* [lecture communication]. Santa Clara, CA: Singularity University.

Cotula, L., Anseeuw, W., & Baldinelli, G. M. (2019). Between promising advances and deepening concerns: A bottom-up review of trends in land governance 2015–2018. *Land, 8*(7), 1–13.

Creswell, J. W. (2014). *Research design: Qualitative, quantitative, and mixed methods approaches* (4th ed.). Thousand Oaks, CA: Sage.

Cueto M. *Medicine and Public Health in Latin America: A History*. New York, NY: Cambridge University Press, 2015.

Dance, G., LaForgia, M., & Confessore, N. (2018). New York Times, December 18th, https://www.nytimes.com/2018/12/18/technology/facebook-privacy.html

De Almeida-Filho N. *La Ciencia Tímida: Ensayos de Deconstrucción de la Epidemiología*. Buenos Aires: Lugar Editorial, 2000.

Donnangelo, M. C. (1976). *Saúde e sociedade*. Sao Paulo, Brazil: Tesis de doutorado, FM/USP.

Donnangelo, M. C. (2014). *O social na epidemiologia em Um legado de Cecília Donnangelo* (J. Carvalheiro, L. Heimann, & M. Derbli, Eds.). São Paulo, Brazil: Instituto de Saúde.

Druker, S. (2013). *Altered genes, twisted truth: How the venture to genetically engineer our food has subverted science, corrupted government and systematically deceived the public*. Salt Lake City, UT: Clear River Press.

Duarte Nunes, E. (1986). *Ciencias Sociales y Salud en la América Latina*. Montevideo, Uruguay: OPS-CIESU.

Dunk, J., Jones, D., Capon, A., & Anderson, W. (2019). Human health on an ailing planet—Historical perspectives on our future. *New England Journal of Medicine, 381*(8), 778–782.

Eastermann, J. (2006). *Filosofía Andina: Sabiduría indígena para un mundo nuevo*. La Paz, Mexico: Central Gráfica.

Echeverría, B. (1990). *La izquierda: Reforma y revolución*. Utopías, Revista de la Facultad de Filosofía y letras–UNAM, 6.

Echeverría, B. (2015). *Siete aproximaciones a Walter Benjamin*. Bogotá, Colombia: Ediciones desde abajo.

Echeverría, B. (2017). *Valor de uso y utopía* (Reprint). Mexico City, Mexico: Siglo Veintiuno.

Eibenschutz, C., Tamez, S., & González, R. (Eds.). (2011). *Determinación social o determinantes sociales de la salud? Memoria del Taller Latinoamericano sobre Determinación Social de la Salud*. Mexico City, Mexico: Universidad Autónoma Metropolitana de Xochimilco.

EJAtlas. (2019). *Environmental justice atlas*. Retrieved from https://ejatlas.org

Equipo Evaluador Internacional. (2017). *Evaluación de la Estrategia Nacional de Inmunizaciones Ecuador 2017*. Quito, Ecuador. Ministerio de Salud Pública/SENPLADES/OPS-OMS, abril.

Erikson, R., & Goldthorpe, J. (1992). *The constant flux: A study of class mobility in industrial societies*. Oxford, UK: Oxford University Press.

Escobar, H. (2019, August 26). There's no doubt that Brazil's fires are linked to deforestation, scientists say. *Science*. Retrieved from https://www.sciencemag.org/news/2019/08/theres-no-doubt-brazils-fires-are-caused-deforestation-scientists-say

Escudero, J. C. (1976). Desnutrición en América Latina (una primera aproximación). *Revista Mexicana de Ciencias Políticas, 84*, 83–130.

Espejo, E. (1930). *Reflexiones sobre el contagio y transmisión de las viruelas por el Doctor Don Francisco Javier Eugenio de Santa Cruz y Espejo*. Quito, Ecuador: Imprenta Municipal. (Original work 1785), 77.

Espejo, E. (1994). *Reflexiones sobre la utilidad, importancia y conveniencias que propone Don Francisco Gil en su disertación físico-médica, acerca de un método seguro para preservar a los pueblos de viruelas*. Quito, Ecuador: Edición facsimilar de la Nueva Editorial de la Casa de la Cultura. Quito, Ecuador: Nueva Editorial de la Casa de la Cultura Ecuatoriana. (Original work published 1785)

Farmer, P. (2005). *Pathologies of power: Health, human rights, and the new war on the poor: With a new preface by the author*. Berkeley, CA: University of California Press.

Felt, U., Fouché, R., Miller, C. A., & Smith-Doerr, L. (Eds). (2017). *The Handbook of Science and Technology Studies*. 4th ed. Cambridge, MA: MIT Press.

Foster, J. B. (2000). *Marx's ecology: Materialism and nature*. New York, NY: Monthly Review Press.

Foucault, M. (1982). The subject and power. In H. L. Dreyfus & P. Rabinow (Eds.), *Michel Foucault. Beyond structuralism and hermeneutics* (pp. 208–226). New York, NY: Harvester Wheatsheaf.

Foucault, M., Lotringer, S., & Hochroth, L. (2007). *The politics of truth*. Los Angeles, CA: Semiotext(e).

Fox, A., & Brainard, J. (2019). University of California takes a stand on open access. *Science, 363*(6431), 1023. Retrieved from https://doi.org/10.1126/science.363.6431.1023-a

Francesca, F. (2013). Posthumanism, transhumanism, antihumanism, metahumanism, and new materialisms: Differences and relations. *Existenz, 8*(2), 26–32.

Franco, S. (2003). A social-medical approach to violence in Colombia. *Am J Public Health, 93*(12), 2032–2036.

Franco, S., Nunes, E., Breilh, J., & Laurell, C. (1991). *Debates in social medicine*. Quito, Ecuador: OPS-ALAMES.

Franco S, Nunes E, Breilh J, Granda E, Yépez, Costales P, Laurell C. *Debates en Medicina Social*. Organizacíon Panamericana de la Salud—Alames. Quito, Ecuador: *Imprenta Non Plus Ultra*, 1991.

Friel S. *Climate Change and The People's Health*. New York, NY: Oxford University Press, 2019.

Fry, R., & Taylor, P. (2013). *A rise for the wealthy; Declines for the lower 93%: An uneven recovery*. Retrieved December 30, 2019, from http://www.pewresearch.org/search/household+recovery

Fukuyama, F. (1989, Summer). The end of history? *The National Interest*, 3–18. ISSN:0884-9382

Galea S, Hernán MA. Win-win: reconciling social epidemiology and causal inference. *Am J Epidemiol* 2019 Oct 3. pii: kwz158. doi: 10.1093/aje/kwz158. [Epub ahead of print]

Galeano, E. (2004). *Las Venas Abiertas de América Latina*. Mexico City, Mexico: Siglo Veintiuno Ediciones.

Garcés, M. (2019). Condición póstuma, o el tiempo del "todo se acaba." *Nueva Sociedad*, *283*, 16–27.

García, C. (1986). *Mortalidad infantil y clases sociales: El caso de Medellín en la década del 70*. Medellín, Colombia: Universidad Pontificia Bolivariana (Ediciones del Cincuentenario).

García, J. C. (1972). *La educación médica en América Latina* (Scientific Publication No. 255). Washington, DC: Organización Panamericana de la Salud/Organización Mundial de la Salud.

García, J. C. (1979). Medicina y sociedad: Ideología y filosofía. In D. Tejeda (Ed.), *Salud y política* (pp. 14–33). Santo Domingo, Dominican Republic: Universidad Autónoma de Santo Domingo.

García Canclini, N. (1993). *Gramsci e as culturas populares na América Latina em "Gramsci e a América Latina"* (C. Coutinho & M. Nogueira, Eds.). São Paulo, Brazil: Paz e Terra.

Grandjean, P., & Landrigan, P. J. (2014). Neurobehavioural effects of developmental toxicity. *Lancet Neurology*, *13*(3), 330–338. Retrieved from https://doi.org/10.1016/S1474-4422(13)70278-3

Guerra, S. (1999). Problemas epistemológicos en el estudio del saber popular. In V. Serrano (Ed.), *Ciencia andina* (pp. 59–72). Quito, Ecuador: Abya Yala/CEDECO.

Habermas, J. (1973). *Teoría analítica de la ciencia y dialéctica en La disputa del positivismo en la sociología* (T. Adorno et al., Eds.). Barcelona, Spain: Grijalbo.

Hahn, N. (2012). The experience of land grab in Liberia. In J. A. Allan, M. Keulertz, S. Sojamo, & J. Warner (Eds.), *Handbook of land and water grabs in Africa—Foreign direct investment and food and water security*. London, UK: Routledge.

Hall, S. (1992). The West and the rest: Discourse and power. In S. Hall & B. Gielben (Eds.), *Formation of modernity* (pp. 276–320). Cambridge, UK: Polity Press/.

Hancock, J. F. (2017). *Plantation crops, plunder and power: Evolution and exploitation*. New York, NY: Routledge.

Harvey, D. (2001). *Spaces of capital: Towards a critical geography*. Edinburgh, UK: Edinburgh University Press.

Harvey, D. (2003). *The new imperialism*. Oxford, UK: Oxford University Press.

Harvey, D. (2007). *Espacios del capital: Hacia una geografía crítica*. Madrid, Spain: Akal Ediciones.

Harvey, D. (2014). *Espacios del capital: Hacia una geografía crítica*. Madrid, Spain: Akal Ediciones.

Hassan, A., Velasquez, E., Belmar, R., Coye, M., Drucker, E., Landrigan, P. J., Michaels, D., & Sidel, K. B. (1981). Mercury poisoning in Nicaragua: a case study of the export of environmental and occupational hazards by a multinational corporation. *Int J Health Services, 11*(2), 221–226.

Herrera, D., González, F., & Saracho, J. F. (2017). *Apuntes teórico-metodológicos para el análisis de la espacialidad: Aproximaciones a la dominación y la violencia. Una perspectiva multidisciplinaria. En Espacio, dominación y violencia*. Mexico City, Mexico: Ediciones Monosílabo–UNAM.

Hill, A. B. (1965). The environment and disease: Association or causation? *Proceedings of the Royal Society of Medicine, 58*(5), 295–300. doi:10.1177/003591576505800503

Holloran, E. (1998). Concepts of infectious disease epidemiology. In K. Rothman & S. Greenland (Eds.), *Modern epidemiology* (pp. 529–554). Philadelphia, PA: Lippincott-Raven.

Hume, D. (1967). *A treatise of human nature*. Oxford, UK: Oxford University Press. (Original work published 1740)

Illich, V. (1966). *Una gran iniciativa en "Obras Escogidas."* Moscow, Russia: Editorial Progreso.

Inman, P., & Smith, H. (2013, June 5). IMF admits: We failed to realise the damage austerity would do to Greece. *The Guardian*. https://www.theguardian.com/business/2013/jun/05/imf-underestimated-damage-austerity-would-do-to-greece

International Peasants Movement. (2008). *La Via Campesina policy documents*. Policy Documents of the 5th Global Congress, Mozambique, Africa.

Ioannidis, J. P. A. (2018). The proposal to lower P value thresholds to .005. *JAMA, 319*(14), 1429–1430.

Iriart, C., Waitzkin, H., Breilh, J., Estrada, A., & Merhy, E. E. (2002). Latin American Social Medicine: contributions and challenges. *Rev Panam Salud Publica*, *12*(2), 128–136.

Irvine, J., Miles, I., & Evans, J. (Eds.). (1979). *Demystifying social statistics*. London, UK: Pluto Press.

Jiménez-Paneque, R. (2016). The questioned *p* value: Clinical, practical and statistical significance. *Medwave*, *16*(8), e6534.

Jones, R., & Wilsdon, J. (2018). *The biomedical bubble. Why UK research and innovation needs a greater diversity of priorities, politics, places and people*. Cambridge, UK: NESTA.

Klein, N. (2000). *No logo*. Toronto, Ontario, Canada: Random House of Canada.

Klein, N. (2007). *The shock doctrine*. Toronto, Ontario, Canada: Random House.

Klein, N. (2008). *La doctrina del shock: El auge del capitalismo del desastre*. Buenos Aires, Argentina: PAIDOS.

Kneen, B. (1999). *Farmageddon: Food and the culture of biotechnology*. Gabriola Island, British Columbia, Canada: New Society Publishers.

Kowii, A. (2011). El Sumak Kawsay. *AportesAndinos*, *28*.

Krieger, N. (1988). Special report—epidemiology in Latin America: the emerging perspective of Social medicine. *Epidemiology Monitor*, *9*, 3–4.

Krieger, N. (1994). Epidemiology and the web of causation: has anyone seen the spider? *Soc Sci Med, 39*, 887–903.

Krieger, N. (2001). Theories for social epidemiology in the 21st century: an ecosocial perspective. *Int J Epidemiol, 30*, 668–677.

Krieger N. Session organizer, "*Latin American Social Medicine and the quest for social justice & public health: linking history, data, and pedagogy,*" 130th annual meeting, American Public Health Association, Philadelphia, PA, Nov 9-13, 2002.

Krieger, N. (2003). Latin American social medicine: the quest for social justice and public health. *Am J Public Health*, *93*(12), 1989–1991.

Krieger N. *Epidemiology and The People's Health: Theory and Context*. New York, NY: Oxford University Press, 2011. (2011a)

Krieger N. Symposium organizer, "*Epidemiologic theories for analyzing health inequities: contributions from Latin America and North America—in global context,*" International Epidemiological Association for the 3rd North American Congress of Epidemiology, Montreal, Quebec, Canada, June 21-24, 2011. (2011b)

Krieger, N. (2014). Got theory?—on the 21st c CE rise of explicit use of epidemiologic theories of disease distribution: a review and ecosocial analysis. *Current Epidemiol Reports, 1*(1), 45–56.

Krieger, N. (2016). Symposium co-organizer, on behalf of the International Epidemiological Association, in collaboration with the American Public Health Association Epidemiology Section, "Epidemiology across the Americas: Connecting Latin American, Caribbean, and North American Epidemiologists to Advance Epidemiological Thinking, Practice, and Health Equity – a panel discussion." *Epidemiology Congress of the Americas,* Miami, FL.

Krieger, N. (2020). Climate crisis, health equity, & democratic governance: the need to act together. *J Public Health Policy.* https://doi.org/10.1057/s41271-019-00209-x (published on-line advance access: January 21, 2020)

Krieger, N. (2005). Embodiment: A conceptual glossary for epidemiology. *Journal of Epidemiology and Community Health, 59,* 350–355. doi:10.1136/jech.2004.024562

Krieger, N. (2011). *Epidemiology and the people's health: Theory and context.* New York, NY: Oxford University Press.

Krieger, N. (2013). *Ecosocial theory of disease distribution: Why epidemiologic theory matters.* Paper presented at the 8th International Seminar on Public Health, March 4, Bogotá, Colombia.

Krieger, N., Alegría, M., Almeida-Filho, N., Barbosa da Silva, J., Barreto, M. L., Beckfield, J., Berkman, L., Birn, A. E., Duncan, B. B., Franco, S., Garcia, D. A., Gruskin, J., James, S. A., Laurell, A. C., Schmidt, M. I., & Walters, K. L. (2010). Who, and what, causes health inequities? Reflections on emerging debates from an exploratory Latin American/North American workshop *J Epidemiol Community Health, 64*(9), 747–749.

Krieger, N., & Davey Smith, G. (2016). The tale wagged by the DAG: broadening the scope of causal inference and explanation for epidemiology. *Int J Epidemiol*, *45*(6), 1787–1808.

Kuhn, T. (1962). *The structure of scientific revolutions*. Chicago, IL: University of Chicago Press.

Kuhn, T. (1970). *The structure of scientific revolutions* (2nd ed.). Chicago, IL: University of Chicago Press.

Kuyek, D. (2001, March). *Intellectual property rights: Ultimate control of R&D in Asia*. Retrieved from https://www.grain.org/article/entries/ 30-intellectual-property-rights-ultimate-control-of-agricultural-r-d-in-asia

Latham, J., Wilson, AK, & Steinbrecher, R. A. (2006). The mutational consequences of plant transformation. *Journal of Biomedicine and Biotechnology*, *2006*, 25376.

Laurell, A. C. (1976). Enfermedad y Desarrollo: Análisis sociológico de la morbilidad en dos pueblos mexicanos. *Revista Mexicana de Ciencias Políticas*, *84*, 131–158.

Laurell, A. C. (1989). Social analysis of collective health in Latin America. *Soc Sci Med*, *28*(11), 1183–1191.

Laurell, A. C. (1994). Sobre la concepción biológica y social del proceso salud enfermedad. In *Desarrollo de recursos humanos: Vol. 101. Lo biológico y lo social: Su articulación en la formación del personal de salud* (pp. 1–12). Washington, DC: OPS.

Laurell, A. C. (2003). What does Latin American social medicine do when it governs? The case of the Mexico City Government. *Am J Public Health*, *93*(12), 2028–2031.

Laurell, A. C. (2018). Lasting Lessons From Social Ideas and Movements of the Sixties on Latin American Public Health. *Am J Public Health*, *108*(6), 730–731.

Latour B. *Down To Earth: Politics in the New Climate Regime*. Cambridge, UK: Polity Press, 2018.

Lawson M, Butt AP, Harvey R, Sarosi D, Coffey C, Piaget K, Tekkudan J. *Time to Care: Unpaid and Underpaid Care Work and the Global Inequality Crisis.*

Oxfam International, 20 January 2020. https://www.oxfam.org/en/research/time-care; accessed: February 12, 2020.

Leavell, H., & Clark, G. (1965). *Preventive medicine for the doctor in his community*. New York, NY: McGraw-Hill.

Lefebvre, H. (1991). *The production of space*. Malden, MA: Blackwell.

Lefebvre, H. (2007). *The production of space*. Malden, MA: Blackwell.

Lefebvre, H. (2014). *Critique of everyday life: The one-volume edition*. New York, NY: Verso.

Leiss, W. (1972). *The domination of nature*. New York, NY: Beacon.

León, M., Jiménez, M., Vidal, N., Bermúdez, K., & De Vos, P. (2020). The role of social movements in strengthening health systems: The experience of the National Health Forum in El Salvador (2009–2018). *International Journal of Health Services, 50*(2), 218–233. Retrieved from https://doi.org/10.1177/0020731420905262

Levins, R., & Lewontin, R. (1985). *The dialectical biologist*: Cambridge, MA: Harvard University Press.

Lukács, G. (2013). *Ontología del ser social: La alienación* (A. Infranca and M. Vedda, Eds.). Buenos Aires, Argentina: Herramienta.

MacMahon, B. (1975). *Principios y métodos de la epidemiología*. Mexico City, Mexico: La Prensa Médica Mexicana.

Marmot, M. G., & Wilkinson, R. G. (Eds.). (2006). *Social determinants of health* (2nd ed.). New York, NY: Oxford University Press.

Marx, K. (1981). *Capital*. New York, NY: Vintage.

Matus, C. (1987). *Adiós Señor Presidente: Planificación, anti-planificación y gobierno*. Caracas, Venezuela: Pomaire.

Melón, D., & Zuberman, F. (Eds.). (2014). *La patria sojera: El modelo agrosojero en el Cono Sur*. Buenos Aires, Argentina: Editorial El Colectivo.

Menéndez, E. (1981). *Poder, estratificación y salud: Análisis de las condiciones sociales y económicas de la enfermedad en Yucatán*. Mexico: Ediciones de la Casa Chata.

Menéndez, E. (1998). Estilos de vida, riesgos y construcción social: Conceptos similares y significados diferentes. *Estudios Sociológicos, 16*(46), 37–67.

Menéndez, E. (2008). Epidemiología sociocultural: Propuestas y posibilidades. *Región y Sociedad, 20*(2). Retrieved from http://www.scielo.org.mx/scielo. php?script=sci_arttext&pid=S1870-39252008000400002

Menéndez, E., & Di Pardo, R. (1996). *De algunos alcoholismos y algunos saberes: Atención primaria y proceso de alcoholización.* Mexico City, Mexico: Centro de Investigación y Estudios Superiores en Antropología Social: Ediciones de La Casa Chata.

Miettinen, O. (1985). *Theoretical epidemiology.* New York, NY: Wiley.

Minayo, C. (1992). *O desafio do conhecimento.* São Paulo, Brazil: HUCITEC-ABRASCO.

Minayo, C. (2009). *La artesanía de la investigación cualitativa.* Buenos Aires, Argentina: Lugar Editorial.

Mining Technology. (2014, April). *Ten technologies with the power to transform mining* [Analysis]. Retrieved from https://www.mining-technology.com/features/featureten-technologies-with-the-power-to-transform-mining-4211240

Ministerio de Salud y Protección Social de Colombia. (2014). *IV Estudio Nacional de Salud Bucal* (Vol. 1: Metodología y Determinación Social de la Salud Bucal; Vol. 2: Situación en Salud Bucal). Bogotá, Colombia: Ministerio de Salud y Protección Social de Colombia.

Morales, C., & Eslava, J. C. (Eds.). (2015). *Tras las huellas de la determinación: Memorias del Seminario Inter-Universitario de Determinación Social de la Salud* (first edition in Spanish). Bogotá, Colombia: Universidad Nacional de Colombia, Sede Bogotá, Facultad de Medicina, Facultad de Odontología.

Morin, E. (2010). *Ciência com consciência.* Rio de Janeiro, Brazil: Bertrand Brasil.

Myers, S. (2018). Planetary health: Protecting human health on a rapidly changing planet. *Lancet, 390,* 2860–2868. doi:10.1016/S0140-6736(17)32846-5

Myers, S. S. (2018). Planetary health: protecting human health on a rapidly changing planet. *Lancet 390*(10114), 2860–2868.

Naughton, J. (2019). To err is human—Is that why we fear machines that can be made to err less? *The Guardian*. Retrieved from https://www.theguardian.com/commentisfree/2019/dec/14/err-is-human-why-fear-machines-made-to-err-less-algorithmic-bias?CMP=share_btn_link

Navarro, V. (2020). A celebration of a half a century's dedication to relevance and scholarship. A note from the founder and Editor-in-Chief, Professor Vicente Navarro. *Int J Health Services*, *50*(1), 5–6.

Nolte, K., Chamberlain, W., & Giger, M. (2016). *International land deals for agriculture: Fresh insights from the Land Matrix: Analytical report II*. Bern, Switzerland: Bern Open Publishing.

Nunes, E. (1996). Saúde Coletiva: Revisitando a sua História e os Cursos de Pós-Graduação. *Saúde Coletiva*, *1*(1), 55–69.

Nuñez, B. (2018). *El Pensamiento Médico de Eugenio Espejo en la Europa del Siglo XVIII*. Quito, Ecuador: Repositorio de la Universidad Andina Simón Bolívar.

Open Markets Institute. (2018). *America's concentration crisis: An Open Markets Institute report*. Retrieved from https://www.openmarketsinstitute.org/publications/americas-concentration-crisis

Oreskes N. *Why Trust Science?* Princeton, NJ: Princeton University Press, 2019.

Otálvaro, G. J. (2019). *Ciudad, juventudes y políticas de salud en Medellín en el siglo XXI*. Quito, Ecuador: Tesis del doctorado en salud, ambiente y sociedad de la Universidad Andina Simón Bolívar.

Otero, G., Pechlaner, G., Liberman, G., & Gürcan, E. (2015). The neoliberal diet and inequality in the United States. *Social Science & Medicine, 142*, 47–55. doi:10.1016/j.socscimed.2015.08.005

Oxford University Press. *Small Books Big Ideas in Population Health*. https://global.oup.com/academic/content/series/s/small-books-big-ideas-in-population-health-sbbi/?lang=en&cc=us; accessed: February 12, 2020.

Paredes, R. (1938). *El imperialismo en el Ecuador: Oro y sangre en Portovelo*. Quito, Ecuador: Editorial Artes Gráficas.

Parsons, T. (1991). *The social system*. London: Routledge.

Passos Nogueira, R. (Ed.). (2010). *Determinação Social da Saúde e Reforma Sanitária*. Rio de Janeiro, Brazil: Centro Brasileiro de Estudos de Saúde (CEBES).

Pauli, B. J. (2019). *Flint fights back: Environmental justice and democracy in the Flint water crisis*. Cambridge, MA: MIT Press.

People's Health Movement. *Global Health Watch 5: An Alternative World Health Report*. London, UK: Zed Books, 2017. https://phmovement.org/download-full-contents-of-ghw5/; accessed: February 12, 2020.

Pew Commission on Industrial Farm Animal Production. (2008). Putting meat on the table: Industrial farm animal production in America. Baltimore, MD: Pew Charitable Trusts and Johns Hopkins Bloomberg School of Public Health.

Phillips, S. (2018, December). Shared mobility by region: South and Latin America [Blog]. Shared mobility thoughts. https://movmi.net/latin-america-shared-mobility/

Piketty, T. (2015). *El capital en el siglo XXI* (E. Cazenave Tapie Isoard & G. Cuevas, Trads.). Mexico City, Mexico: Ediciones Fondo de Cultura Económica.

Popay, J. (2003). Qualitative research and the epidemiological imagination: A vital relationship. *Gaceta Sanitaria, 17*(Suppl. 3), 65.

Punch, K. (2014). *Introduction to social research: Quantitative and qualitative approaches*. Thousand Oaks, CA: Sage.

Punch, K. (2016). *Developing effective research proposals* (3rd ed.). Thousand Oaks, CA: Sage.

Reese, A. (2006). *Genetically modified food: A short guide for the confused*. London, UK: Pluto Press.

Ribeiro, S. (2016). *Cuarta revolución industrial, tecnologías en impactos*. El Ciervo Herido, Blog of Omar González. Retrieved from https://elciervoherido.wordpress.com/2016/11/21/cuarta-revolucion-industrial-tecnologias-e-impactos-silvia-ribeiro

Robinson WR, Bailey ZD. What social epidemiology brings to the table: reconciling social epidemiology and causal inference. *Am J Epidemiol* 2019 Sep 30. pii: kwz197. doi: 10.1093/aje/kwz197. [Epub ahead of print]

Rodríguez-Beltrán, C. (2018). *Principios de la inteligencia artificial*. Paper presented at the Conferencia al Seminario Internacional "Nuevas Tendencias Tecnológicas y sus Impactos en América Latina," Mexico City, Mexico, May 21.

Rogers, A., Woodward, A., Swinburn, B., & Dietz, W. (2018, April). Prevalence trends tell us what did not precipitate the US obesity epidemic. *Lancet Public Health, 3*(4), e153.

Roig, A. A. (2013). *Esquemas para una historia de la filosofía ecuatoriana* (3rd ed., Vol. 22). Quito, Ecuador: Corporación Editora Nacional.

Rorty, R. (1994). *Habermas y Lyotard sobre la posmodernidad en "Habermas y la Modernidad* (R. Berstein, Ed.; pp. 253–276). Madrid, Spain: Editorial Cátedra.

Rosen, G. (1958). *A history of public health.* New York, NY: MD Publications.

Rosset, P., & Altieri, Mi. (2019). Agroecología: Ciencia y política (A. Porras, Trad.; 1era ed.). MAPorrúa.

Rothman, K. J., & Greenland, S. (1998). *Modern epidemiology* (2nd ed.). Philadelphia: Lippincott—Raven.

Sackett, D. (2000). The sins of expertness and a proposal for redemption. *British Medical Journal, 320*(7244), 1283.

Samaja, J. (1997). *Epistemología y metodología: Elementos para una teoría de la investigación.* Buenos Aires, Argentina: EUDEBA.

Samaja, J. (2005). *Epistemología y metodología: Elementos para una teoría de la investigación científica* (3rd ed.). Buenos Aires, Argentina: EUDEBA.

Sánchez Parga, J. (2011). Discursos retrovolucionarios: Sumak Kawsay, derechos de la naturaleza y otros pachamamismos. *Ecuador Debate, 84,* 31–50.

Santos, B. de S. (2014). *Epistemologies of the South: Justice against epistemicide.* New York, NY: Paradigm.

Santos, M. (1985). *Espaço e método.* Sao Paulo, Brazil: Nobel.

Santos, M. (1996). *A natureza do espaço: Técnica e tempo; Razão e emoção.* São Paulo, Brazil: Editora Hucitec.

Schwartz, S., Gatto, N. M., & Campbell, U. B. (2016). Causal identification: a charge of epidemiology in danger of marginalization. *Am J Epidemiol, 26*(10), 669–673.

Siegel, S. (2013). *EIA interview with Shefa Siegel on "The Missing Ethics of Mining."* Retrieved November 22, 2015, from http://www.ethicsandinternationalaffairs.org/2013/5340

Sigerist, H. (1945). *Civilization and disease*. Ithaca, NY: Cornell University Press.

Smith, L. T. (1999). *Decolonizing methodologies: Research and indigenous peoples*. New York, NY: Zed Books.

Solíz, F. (2016). *Salud colectiva y ecología política: La basura en Ecuador*. Quito, Ecuador: Universidad Andina Simón Bolívar, Ediciones la Tierra.

Solíz Torres, M. F. (2018). *Fruta del norte: La manzana de la discordia: Monitoreo comunitario participativo y memoria colectiva en la comunidad de El Zarza*. Quito, Ecuador: Universidad Andina Simón Bolívar, Ediciones la Tierra.

Stoll, L., Michaelson, J., & Seaford, C. (2012). *Well-being evidence for policy*. London, UK: New Economics Foundation.

Straffon, A. (2018). *Impactos de la geoingeniería del manejo de la radiación solar*. Paper presented at the Conferencia al Seminario Internacional "Nuevas Tendencias Tecnológicas y sus Impactos en América Latina," Mexico City, Mexico, May 21.

Subirats, J. (2019). ¿Del poscapitalismo al postrabajo? *Nueva sociedad*, *279*, 34–48.

Tajer, D. (2003). Latin American social medicine: roots, development during the 1990s, and current challenges. *Am J Public Health*, *93*(12), 2023–2027.

Tambellini, A. M. (1978). *O trabalho e a doença em "Saúde e medicina no Brasil: Contribução para um debate."* Rio de Janciro, Brazil: GRAAL.

Tashakkori, A., & Teddlie, C. (1998). *Combining qualitative and quantitative approaches* (Applied social research methods series, Vol. 46). London, UK: Sage.

Tesh, S. (1988). *Hidden arguments: Political ideology and disease prevention policy*. New Brunswick, NJ: Rutgers University Press.

Thompson, J. (2010). A taxonomy of interdisciplinarity. In R. Frodeman, J. Thompson, & C. Mitcham (Eds.), *The Oxford handbook of interdisciplinarity* (pp. 15–30). Oxford, UK: Oxford University Press.

Uding, N., & Schreder, E. (2015). *Chemicals revealed: Over 5000 kids' products contain toxic chemicals*. Seattle, WA: Toxic Free Future/Washington Toxics Coalition.

United Kingdom Department of Health and Social Security. (1982). *Inequalities in health: The Black report*. London, UK: Penguin.

242   REFERENCES

United Nations, Department of Economic and Social Affairs, Population Division. (2017a). *International migration report 2017: Highlights* (ST/ESA/SER.A/404). New York, NY: Author.

United Nations, Special Rapporteur on the Right to Food. (2017b, January 24). *Report to the general assembly* (A/HRC/34/48, p. 4). New York, NY: Author.

Vandenbroucke, J. P., Broadbent, A., & Pearce, N. (2016). Causality and causal inference in epidemiology: the need for a pluralistic approach. *Int J Epidemiol*, *45*(6), 1776–1786.

VanderWeele T. *Explanation in Causal Inference: Methods for Mediation and Interaction*. New York: Oxford University Press, 2015.

Vasquez, E. E., Perez-Brumer, A., & Parker, R. G. (2019). Social inequities and contemporary struggles for collective health in Latin America. *Global Public Health*, *14*(6–7), 777–790.

Victora, C., Barros, F. C., & Vaughan, J. P. (1992). *Epidemiologia de la desigualdad: Un estudio longitudinal de 6,000 niños brasileños*. Washington, DC: Organización Panamericana de la Salud, Oficina Sanitaria Panamericana, Oficina Regional de la Organización Mundial de la Salud.

Vidal, J., & Guest, P. (2015, August 15). How developing countries are paying a high price for the global mineral boom. *The Guardian*. Retrieved from https://www.theguardian.com/global-development/2015/aug/15/developing-countries-high-price-global-mineral-boom

Virchow, R. (1848). Report on the typhus epidemic in Upper Silesia. *Medical Reform*, 8.

Waitzkin H. *Medicine and Public Health at the End of Empire*. Boulder, CO: Paradigm Publishers, 2011.

Waitzkin, H. (2011). *Medicine and public health at the end of empire*. New York, NY: Paradigm.

Waitzkin, H., Iriart, C., Buchanan, H. S., Mercado, F., Tregear, J., & Eldrege, J. (2008). The Latin American Social Medicine Database: a resource for epidemiology. *Int J Epidemiol*, *37*(4), 724–728.

Waitzkin, H., Iriart, C., Estrada, A., & Lamadrid, S. (2001). Social medicine then and now: lessons from Latin America. *Am J Public Health*, *91*(10), 1592–601.

Waitzkin, H., Iriart, C., Estrada, A., & Lamadrid, S. (2001). Social medicine in Latin America: Productivity and dangers facing the major national groups. *Lancet*, *358*(9278), 315–323.

Waitzkin, H., & the Working Group for Health Beyond Capitalism (Eds.). (2018). *Health care under the knife: Moving beyond capitalism for our health*. New York, NY: Monthly Review Press.

Weber, M. (1978). *Economy and society*. Berkeley, CA: University of California Press.

World Health Organization. (2019). *Social determinants of health*. Retrieved from https://www.who.int/social_determinants/thecommission/en

Wright, E. O. (Ed.). (2005). *Approaches to class analysis*. Cambridge, UK: Cambridge University Press.

Wright, S. (1994). *Molecular politics: Developing American and British policy for genetic engineering, 1972–1982*. Chicago, IL: University of Chicago Press.

Wu, T. (2018). *The curse of bigness: Antitrust in the new gilded age*. New York, NY: Columbia Global Reports.

Yamada, S. (2003). Latin American social medicine and global social medicine. *Am J Public Health, 93*, 1994–1996.

Ziman, J. (2002). *Real science: What it is, and what it means*. Cambridge, UK: Cambridge University Press.

INDEX

For the benefit of digital users, indexed terms that span two pages (e.g., 52–53) may, on occasion, appear on only one of those pages.

Tables and figures are indicated by *t* and *f* following the page number

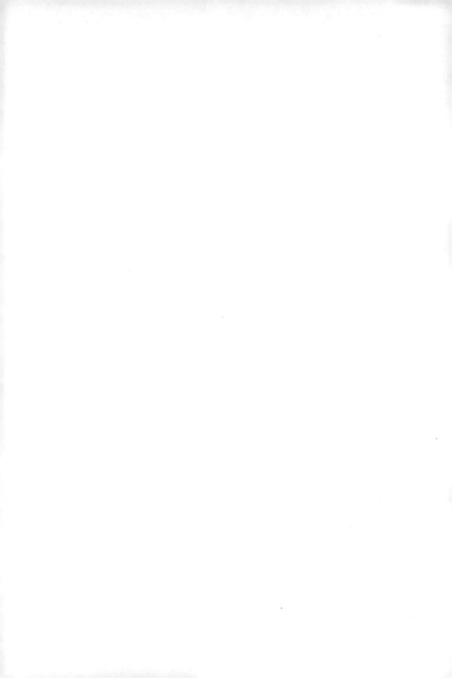